Never Say

Never

To Tracy & Linda

Compelling Story

ISBN #-10:1984331256

Published 2018

Doris Schultz Cowfer

Clarence D. Cowfer (Dave)

Acknowledgements

Thanks to Joy Thomas for editing and outstanding support, making publication of this book possible.

Thanks to the Aiken, South Carolina community churches, friends, and family for their prayers and over 400 get well cards we received during our 14 weeks in Florida after Doris' tragic fall.

Special thanks to Dr. Jacobs' Neuro-Surgical team, the Shands Hospital at The University of Florida, and Brookes Rehab Hospital, Jacksonville, FL. The Shands and Brookes Rehab teams made it possible for a Gross Motor Quadriplegic to regain motor functions to the extent her spinal cord injury would allow. The Brookes Rehab team taught me how to care for Doris.

Thanks to our local Aiken/Augusta Medical/Rehab doctors and hospitals, especially National Health Care Rehab and Nursing facility in North Augusta, making it possible for us to enjoy Doris for 8 wonderful years after her SCI.

Thanks to Doris our rock star, the most courageous and dedicated SCI patient on the planet. Thanks, and praise be to God for the miracle of Doris and me focusing solely on each other for 8 years. I shall treasure it to my grave.

Dedication

To Doris Schultz Cowfer, an inspiration to all. Faced with life-changing challenges, she met life's biggest challenge head-on on January 4th, 2006.

FOREWORD

"It was a beautiful sunny day in Florida... I saw a planting of pansies... with some dead ones on it... I did not know if he (my son) knew that he should pinch them back, you know take the dead ones off. "

So much like Doris.

The events that followed created the greatest challenges Dave and Doris would ever face in life.

The harrowing, frightening medical and personal drama that unfolded when Doris bent forward, as she did not want to get her new pants dirty when she did a bit of gardening, poignantly shows the character of a true lady that understood the fall she had taken forever changed her life. She did not panic, as she never did during the next eight years, always thinking about how to overcome one obstacle after another.

Doris encouraged Dave to go to a Penn State football games and occasionally use his fly rod, all the time facing personal and medical challenges, unanticipated complications of medical therapy and, finally, facing an insurmountable life ending challenge of leukemia.

Doris and Dave described the many problems faced by people with cervical spinal cord injuries, the many problems encountered in making efforts at finding the best available care in a timely manner and the many physicians, nurses, administrators, technicians that a person encounters and the impact that each makes on an individual who is vulnerable to even the most inconsequential expression of frustration misdirected.

Doris had a caring partner who sought out the very best he knew to help his wife. Every time a problem arose, as it inevitably does in the chronic care of a person with a spinal cord injury, Dave found a solution.

Doris and Dave described the experiences with the many institutions, and people who helped Doris gain as much as recovery as she could.

Ossified posterior longitudinal ligament and a little pansy patch so much changed the lives of these wonderful and personally committed friends, partners, spouses.

Read about the experiences Doris had and endured until the ultimate unsolvable problem took her life. This book should be an encouragement to all facing obstacles that seem insurmountable. The emotion of the minute should be understood by all who provide help to those spinal cord injured, so vulnerable, so in need. Doris is fortunate to have had Dave. We are fortunate to have known both.

Gerald Gordon, MD FACP

PREFACE

This book is Doris' message to ladies with Osteoarthritis and/or a cervical spine condition called "Ossified Posterior Longitudinal Ligament".

On January 4th, 2006, Doris noticed some dead pansies in our son's flower bed on the way to retrieve the morning paper. She stopped to "deadhead' the pansies and, as she bent over from the waist, she fell on her chin and lay there paralyzed from the shoulders down. Compression fractures in a ligament surrounding her spinal cord in her neck that, over time from arteritis and lack of calcium in her body, had become boney-like and very brittle. These compression fractures penetrated her spinal cord from cervical vertebra C3 down to just below the base of her neck to T1 paralyzing her.

Doris did not panic. A woman of utmost faith had a conversation with God, as you will see in her own words in Chapter One. She could speak and shout for help. When help arrived, she started to determine why she could not move. She asked our daughter-in-law to help her determine if she had had a stroke, giving Pat step by step instructions on what to do. Her message simply put is, "Ladies, when gardening or picking something off the floor, never bend from the waist or never lead with your chin". Bend or squat at the knees. Never put yourself in a position to fall on your face. Doris' message and story detailed in this book are intended to make you aware of the risks of falling and provide information useful to you if, God forbid, you become paralyzed in a fall.

Any recovery from an SCI, if possible, depends upon the proper care administered at the time of the injury. EMS, ER, and the skills of the Corrective Surgery Team are critical. The patient's attitude and trust that physical and other therapies will produce results is paramount. Doris' spectacular achievements from the neck down paralysis at the moment of her fall to accomplish a life in a wheelchair shows vivid proof that rehab works. I must add that physical therapy brought her back to transferring in and out of her wheelchair, six to eight recoveries per year for at least seven years from extended hospitalizations. Follow-up medical, recovery and rehab teams enable a willing patient to recover what mobility the extent of his/her injuries will allow.

Doris had the best available SCI care on the East Coast in 2006. The ER and ICU teams at Orange Park Hospital performed their initial treatment and care for six days awaiting transfer to a University Level Trauma Team. The Neural Surgical Team at the University of Florida headed by Dr. Jacobs performed an outstanding job. Brookes Rehab in Jacksonville and follow up at outpatient Walton Rehab in Augusta brought her back to transferring in and out of her power wheelchair. She progressed to walking short distances with a walker and an attendee holding on to her. An amazing recovery over a four-month period. As her 24/7 caregiver apart from feeding, administering meds, toileting, bathing, physically positioning her for comfort and dressing, my job was to monitor wellness by symptoms and respond to them as needed. I was not going to lose my Doris to any illness we could do something about. My career as a scientist and my mechanical bent helped tremendously. I learned a lot and the joy of working one-on-one with Doris was the most rewarding time of my life.

Once Doris got through the initial corrective surgery and proceeded to inpatient rehab, it took me two to three months to realize that Doris' motor functions had completely disengaged from her brain memory. Witnessing what she had to endure to teach her brain to perform what motor functions she was physically able to recover, was the most uplifting and courageous experience of my life. Initially, I rejoiced at the first leg movement, or any movement she could do that was requested by her therapists. Simple leg movement convinced me she was on the way to full recovery. I could not have been more wrong.

We left home in Aiken, SC the last week of December and returned mid-April in a new Wheelchair Access Handicap Van. Doris' eight-year survival was a 24/7 process made possible by a team including Dr. Gerald Gordon her personal physician, a noted Infections Specialist. Continued infections care is essential for survival for SCI patients with limited mobility compounded, as in Doris' case, with a neurogenic bladder. We lived each day realizing we were dealing with a life-threatening situation.

The first two chapters in this book are Doris' own words describing her tragic fall and quadriplegia living eight years in a wheelchair combating a multitude of health care issues. Doris' demeanor and attitude from the moment of her fall and immediate paralysis will blow your mind. She epitomized the power of prayer and utmost faith enabling her inner nature to work miracles in this crisis and many others she/we experienced in our fifty-eight years of marriage. She especially wanted to warn women with Osteoarthritis and other cervical spine ossification conditions of the dangers they face in the simplest of falls. She believed spinal cord injury SCI patients could learn from her experience because the uniqueness of each and every injury and prognosis on recovery is not possible. She dearly wanted to go to military hospitals to show brain and spinal cord patients that they could accomplish what a 69-year-old lady did.

SECTION ONE

Doris' dictated report of her tragic fall
and paralysis on January 4, 2006

It was a beautiful sunny day in Florida where we were visiting our son and family. I got up and put on my newest Christmas outfit, one that I loved: slacks and a red sweater, my favorite color. When I went downstairs, no one was up yet so I decided to go get the Sunday paper.

They have a long driveway, and on the way down the drive, I saw a planting of pansies with some dead ones on it. My son does the landscaping around their house and I did not know if he knew that he should pinch them back; you know, take the dead ones off. I decided I would bend over and deadhead the pansies. I did not want to put my knees on the ground because I had on my new slacks, so I bent over.

All of a sudden, the ground became closer and closer but I was not dizzy. The next thing I knew (I don't know how long I may have lain there; my granddaughter thinks it was only a few minutes), I couldn't understand why I couldn't lift my arm. I could see it but not lift it.

My son mulches his beds thickly, so I am trying hard with my tongue to get the pine straw or the mulch out of my mouth. I know I swallowed a little so I prayed to the Lord and said, *Lord, you are going to have to help me out of this because I do not know what has happened.*

I could not move, other than being able to turn my head a little. As I say, I was trying to get the mulch out of my mouth so I could yell for help. I finally got enough out that I could start yelling because people walk in that neighborhood. The house sits back from the road so I did not think anyone would hear me. Unfortunately, as well, I landed with my head turned toward the house.

Every so often I would yell, "Help", and again, a car went by, a pickup went by, and I'm still yelling, "Help me, I think I may have had a stroke," because I didn't know of any other explanations for not being able to move.

The next thing I knew, I was looking at the great big feet of a dog and a pair of tennis shoes.

I said, "Oh, dear God, thank you for sending me this woman.

She said, "I always carry my cell phone and today I didn't. I'm not familiar with this neighborhood; I walk through it, but I don't live here."

I said, "Well, go up and get in the garage door and when you get in the house, you'll see a phone, a portable phone, on the wall and you can bring it."

She left, but soon came back and said, "I can't get in the garage door."

Well, I should have said the door by the garage door; I knew it was open because I just came out of it. Then, God love her, she went back and did that.

I said, "You can call for my daughter-in-law, her name is Pat. You can call for her; she has a back bedroom,"

Anyway, it was more important that she get out of the house with the phone.

When she got back, she was so nervous, and she said, "I don't know how I can help you." She said, "I'm calling 911."

She didn't know the street name or number and had to go back into the house to find my daughter-in-law Pat who, by that time, was in the kitchen and had thought she'd heard somebody come in. The young woman told my daughter-in-law that I was lying in the yard so Pat came out and they called 911 and gave them the address.

My dear Pat lay down on the ground with me and started trying to get some of the mulch out of my mouth. My glasses were still on.

I said, "Are my glasses broken?"

She said, "No, they're fine, but I have to get some of this mulch out of them."

I knew I couldn't see well. It was stuck in my glasses and I guess my hair was full of it.

Anyway, she was trying to do that and I said, "Pat, I'm going to smile and if my mouth goes crooked, tell me. I smiled but my mouth didn't go crooked. I said, "Now I'm going to stick my tongue out. If it pulls to the left or the right, tell me."

Well, I stuck my tongue out and she said, "No, it didn't."

I said, "Well, I thought maybe I'd had a stroke because I can't feel anything." I said, "Are my legs sticking up in the air?"

She said, "No, they're flat on the ground."

At that point, EMS and the police were there surveying everything. They told Pat to go get a spray bottle of water so she could get the mulch out of my mouth. Then, they debated how to get me out of this position. In retrospect, they did not do it right.

I mean, I remember the police officer saying, "We'll just pick her up and put her on the stretcher."

They should have put the board on my back, but first should have put a neck brace on me because I'd told them I couldn't feel anything from my neck down. They debated and debated and, finally, they just laid the board on the ground next to me and essentially flipped me over and lifted me into the ambulance.

My daughter-in-law followed to the small Orange Park Hospital. All ER rooms were full, so they had seven of us in the hall. Once in the ambulance when the shock wore off I was in excruciating pain shooting down across my shoulders and down both arms. It was the worst pain I ever experienced; I can't even describe it.

During the ambulance ride, the EMS person had called in and said that they were bringing me in with what appeared to be a spinal injury. They did a simple test but I couldn't feel it in my arms and legs, or chest.

He started counting down, talking to me … "It is 20 minutes to the hospital Mrs. Cowfer; now 15 minutes, 10 minutes, just hold on, hold on."

Then the driver said, "I think you should put a neck brace on her." The attendant finally did put a neck brace on me. I don't know that they did any damage; the damage had probably already occurred, I feel sure.   But they should have taken precautions and put a neck brace on me immediately.

When we got to the hospital, like I say, there were seven of us in the hall, and by that time, the pain was so bad I asked my daughter-in-law, who was there with me, "Honey, take my rings off before my hands start to swell," and she got them off.

The nurse evaluated me but she said the neurosurgeon was in the operating room and she couldn't do anything without his approval. Well, I endured the pain I don't know how long and finally told my daughter-in-law, "Go get that nurse and tell her she's got to give me something for pain because I can't take it anymore. I'm afraid I'm going to start screaming." She went to the nurse and told her and, I don't recall if she gave me something or not.

My husband and son had been at the Orange Bowl and were on their way home. Pat had told our granddaughter, who was fourteen or fifteen at the time, to call her dad on his cell phone. She did call, and my husband was driving when our son told him that someone found me lying in the yard appearing paralyzed.

Well, my husband started speeding he was so worried, so my son said to him, "Dad, I don't think this is the time for you to drive; pull over and I will drive."

Anyway, they finally got there and I was still in the hall. At that point, the neurosurgeon came down. I guess they must have given me something for pain and it was helping a little bit but not much. He ordered more pain medication, put an IV in, and sent me for a CAT Scan. Very shortly after, he was back and told my husband and me that I had terrible damage to my neck.

He said, "It looks like it's from C-3 to T-1." He continued, "Her neck is a mess. If it is repairable, it can only be done at a university-level hospital. I know the doctor who can do it. He's at Shands Hospital in Gainesville, at the University of Florida."

I mean, if I had to have this happen, it was better to have happened in Florida than in my backyard in South Carolina, because I could have laid there forever. Well, a long time, not forever, but I finally got from the hallway into an ER room sometime in the night. That's a long time when you consider I fell at 8:30 that morning.

I don't know how many days went by. I think four or five, but the neurosurgeon did the proper thing in Orange Park. It is so important with a spinal cord injury to keep the inflammation down, and so the procedure is to start heavy, heavy dosages of IV steroids. They did get me started on the steroids, needed within so many hours, although it was borderline by the time they got the doctor down there and had the CAT Scan. Getting me ready for the CAT Scan was quite an adventure.

It stands to reason, they could not move me much, so they cut off all my clothes and it broke my heart. They were brand new and on me for just a few hours, my beautiful slacks and sweater. Our son bought me the sweater; it was red. He always buys me a red sweater and it was so pretty. I said, "Do you have to?" We had two nurses, one on each side, cutting off my clothes.

I lay there, I think, four days; because they couldn't get in contact with the Gainesville surgeon, the one the Orange Park doctor wanted me to have. He went to medical school with him. The Orange Park neurosurgeon was well known. We learned that other neurosurgeons went to him when they had neck problems. But he said mine was too complicated, so he wanted the Shands Hospital Gainesville doctor to do it. Bottom line is they had several days of phone tag and no contact. I suspect that, because they were friends and he was a very busy neurosurgeon, he didn't return calls he might have considered friendship chat calls.

The word got around quickly that my son's mother had fallen in his front yard and was paralyzed. Well, I really did not fall but, anyway, during a conversation with a friend who came to our son's office and inquired about me he said, "If we could just get a hold of the darn doctor." He explained that "That's what's holding everything up; we can't get a hold of this neurosurgeon. "

Then He told her the surgeon's name and she said, "My sister is his secretary."

He said, "Well, let's get her on the phone."

Well, they did and the wheels started turning. It was late at night by the time arrangements were made for me to go to Shands Hospital in Gainesville. The ambulance people who came to get me complained about why they always seemed to get the night shift and blah, blah, blah. I was so thankful that I was going to Shands, but the driver had never driven there and the girl sitting in the back with me had been there but it was probably 10 pm, midnight, I'm not sure. It was a several hours' drive, maybe 3 or 4 hours, I don't know. And, good heavens, he hit every railroad crossing and it was not much of a cot in the ambulance. I felt every bump, and then he got lost. The ride was a nightmare.

They had given me an enormous shot of painkiller before I left the hospital for the ride, and the driving and turning and getting lost a couple of times made me sick, so I started getting nauseated. Anyway, we made it and they took me directly to pre-op. I laid there with a whole line of people; of course, some were going to different operating rooms. The room they needed for me was a special operating room. I finally went into surgery about 7 PM.

They did whatever they could for me to keep me comfortable but nothing really worked. My son and husband placed their warm hands at the base of my neck, under my fractures, it helped because they could not sedate me with surgery pending. To make a long story short, I don't know how long I lay there. It may have been 5 hours or more before the doctor was available. When they finally took me to the operating room, there was a resident there, the one that had checked me out on arrival and in pre-op. The room was completely stainless steel. I'm lying on a stainless-steel slab and the one just above me is identical to the one beneath me.

I said to the resident, "I'm going to have to be on my stomach to have this surgery, aren't I?"

He said, "Yes, ma'am, you are."

I said, "How do I get there?"

He said, "You see that thing above you?"

I said, "Yes."

He said, "Well, once we get you ready to go, we will bring that down like a sandwich and turn you over onto it; the whole thing turns automatically."

He was doing whatever he had to do and the next thing I know, I don't think it was the surgeon; probably the anesthesiologist who said, "Are you ready to get rid of this pain?"

I said, "Oh please, whatever you can do." That's the last thing I remember until I was in another room and the doctor came in to tell me that I was a quadriplegic.

The next morning, I was still on steroids. My husband stayed right by the bed; he had not slept for a couple of days. My son finally convinced him to go to a hotel up the street and get some rest, saying that he could walk back to the hospital the next morning. When he got back to the hospital the next morning (this was actually 2 weeks later in real time), there was a slight movement of the right index finger of my left hand, just a tiny little bit. That was the first movement that I made. We praised God and rejoiced in the success of the surgery.

After I had my surgery in Shands … they had me hooked up to all kinds of sensors. The alarms kept going off on my heart sensor. My heart rate was going down into the thirties; my blood pressure was in the 80s, which is dangerous. I thought these were life-threatening times. They (Shands Heart Team) wanted to check out my heart because they concluded that the low heart rate may have made me fall. They also wanted to do the heart study to see if an irregular heart rate may have caused my fall. Shands is a heart transplant hospital so we agreed to the catheter lab study. When we returned home, my cardiologist was upset that they put me through a study because of my Quad state. I did not have an irregular heartbeat. I had a nurse with me at all times, maybe two, and when they were injecting adrenalin through IV into my heart, I went into atrial fibrillation and they had to shock my heart back into rhythm with the paddles. Not a good experience.

SECTION TWO

Doris' continued dictation recording her experiences in initial rehab at Shands Hospital, Brooks Rehab Hospital in Jacksonville and the many rehab experiences she endured after coming home for the time period

Hours after my surgery, while I was still on high pain medication, a physical therapist (PT) visited me. I was surprised to see that the PT, a young woman who did the initial fitness observation, was also a paraplegic. She was in a small wheelchair and she started feeling my muscle tone all over my arms and legs. She scooted around the bed doing a very thorough examination. I assume she came up with an evaluation because the next day two PT gals came to my room and said they were going to sit me up (this was over a 5-7-day schedule).

I couldn't believe that was going to be a possibility, but they started, and they wrapped both legs with tape and one got behind me to hold me up because I couldn't sit up and they wanted me to dangle for a few minutes. I did get dizzy and was exhausted, so they slowly put me back to bed or laid me down, I should say. Every day they moved me and I'm not sure how long that went on. Eventually, when I was ready, they discharged me to a rehab hospital called Brooks Rehab in Jacksonville, Florida. I had requested to go back to Jacksonville so it would be easier for my family, and my husband could stay with the family and not have to stay in a hotel.

Brooks Rehab is what saved my life. It gave me a reason to believe that I could do something. It was very deliberate and long, hard work. You had three hours in the morning; you had a lunch break; and three hours in the afternoon. I was very lucky to have my case sent to PT. They met and called the head of PT; I think her name was Sarah. She had been there since the day the doors opened. She had worked there 32 years. She was a black lady and I learned to love her. She was so helpful.

Another fortunate thing that happened is a student aide who was there the first two weeks that I was there. I was put into a wheelchair in a sling by an overhead lift. I really don't know how they managed to get me on the mat, but she stood behind me and pushed me up, holding me there as the young man started at my toes. He moved each toe, moving up the leg, following every nerve, every muscle. I tired easily so they let me rest often. Then, they would repeat it again.

This went on for a couple of days until they had really worked very hard on strengthening my legs. So, it may have been a week, I'm not sure, but they decided that they were going to try to stand me up. They wrapped my legs very tight.

I said, "Why do you that?"

She said, "It's because a lot of people pass out when they first stand up."

They used two pieces of equipment to help people stand the first time. Unfortunately, the newest version was in use. Therefore, I had the old sling and straps version, which was a sling they put me in … how I don't know. I don't remember that at all. I think it was by hand that they pulled me up there; it was like a desk type thing at the top and when I got there they told me to try to hold on to the edge of the table. Well, I don't know how long it lasted, it didn't last long. However, they were satisfied that I had been able to do it even though I had not remembered the pain associated with it. And the fear.

There is terrible fear when they put you in those machines and do things with you. You don't know what's going to happen. This one went for a few days and I was finally able to sit with some assistance. They would get me dangled on the edge of the pad so that they could let go of my back, and as the rehab went on, that was the first machine I used and we probably did that for a week. Time eludes me. Then they would put me in my wheelchair between the parallel bars, and stand me up. She would sit on a small stool with wheels in front of me and try to make me walk. I can't remember how they strapped in my upper arms; obviously, they had, because I could get my arms up on those rails.

The first time I only took a couple of steps. But we worked on that every day. She would lift my left foot, then the right foot, but before that, she had me pat my feet. If you've ever seen a baby trying to stand or start to walk, they always stamp their feet on the floor. That's exactly what she had me doing. I guess I did that first, just stamping my feet, and then each day a little more and before long, that's when she had me standing and trying to walk. I really didn't have feeling but yet she was having me stamp left, right, left right, and then she would take her hands off my legs and ask me to keep doing it and I could only take a step or two and I couldn't move it any further.

She would say, "Look down," and here my right foot would be on top of my left foot. She had to work with that; it is proprioception. She never gave up on me and, in fact, several of the PT's came over and clapped the first day that I walked most of the length of the way along the bars with her in front of me, of course with everyone watching me; it was funny.

Then I graduated to other machines. A bicycle type thing that I operated from my wheelchair, to strengthen my legs, and again, pulling me up into a standing position again. We were just getting some strength in my legs and strength in my arms so I could use the parallel bars. I was there for about three months and it was 6 hours a day of treatment. My PT person seemed to be the head person; well I know she was. She would let OT (Occupational Therapy) work with me.

The role of the occupational therapist(OT) was to work on my upper body, where PT worked on my lower body. He was a nice young man, and he did all the arm exercises. It was impossible to unclench my hands so that I could hold onto the parallel bars. I don't know how they managed to get my hands on the parallel bars, but his main job was to get my hands to be usable and to strengthen my upper body.

There were many machines that I used, his working with heat and cold, and every muscle in my arm trying to get my hands to open. It turned out that I had to have OT in the afternoons, PT in the mornings and as hard as he tried, the hands did not do well. After many weeks, I worked on a machine they called "ground up cornhusks," which was heated, and I slid my arms through a rubber gasket. The reason they called it ground up cornhusks was that your arms had to slide through the rubber gasket. That was to warm up the arm and to make it easier to work with.

After maybe a month went by, a sales representative came with new equipment that was supposed to do wonders for people who could not open their hands.

My OT person said, "Doris, I think you're ready for this. Let's go over and see. I think you're a candidate for this."

Well, unfortunately, there was another man using the left-hand equipment so he used the right-hand equipment on me. Actually, the salesperson did it. And he got it into my right hand and I don't know what happened, if it was on too long or if he gave me too much of a zap because it was an electrical stimulus, but my fingers did start to open but, unfortunately, then they couldn't get them closed. It made my right-hand look usable but it wasn't. I can push stuff with it but I can't hold anything, and since it's my right hand, my brain seems to tell me to pick up things with my left hand and try to put it in my right hand and, of course, I always drop it because it doesn't close.

So, using the new machine to open my hand was a real mistake. My arm nerves were not firing enough to respond to the computer. They aborted the test, but my right hand stayed open and could not close. I spent many hours in therapy attempting to develop a grip and use of my right hand, it never happened. We continued to work with strengthening my upper body which I found later was a big help for me because with no feeling in my legs they got my arms strong enough that I could hold on to the bars better and would be able to walk better.

My routine was every morning the aides would rush, rush, rush to get me bathed and I had to wear pants. I couldn't wear dresses in the rehab room because there were males there, too, and certain exercises weren't conducive to wearing a dress or a skirt. One reason we had to wear pants was that is how they gripped you. They didn't really want to grip your arms or legs or any place on your body so they would grab your pants to try to make you stand up. There were many machines, many bicycles that I could operate from my wheelchair for OT. Every day, I did the parallel bars and still had to watch constantly about one foot stepping on the other foot. I finally seemed to conquer that. The brain started working I guess.

What she did for me was unbelievable. She was my head PT person and she wouldn't let anybody else touch me. To think that I went into that rehab the first day that I could not sit up by myself. It was a long journey. In order to sit up and gain strength in my upper arms, I had to use many machines with countless people working, on my arms and hands. I'll never forget Sarah. She was a Godsend for me. She was sick one day. She had requested a certain PT to work with me who came over and said, "Doris, look at this." It was a page of very fine written detailing what she could do and what she couldn't do. Sarah emphasized this PT to not try to walk me. She only trusted herself to do that. So, this substitute PT would put my wheelchair up to the pedals on a bike machine set up for different functions or stuff for strengthening. She turned it over to OT and they did their thing, which consisted of hot and cold compresses, mostly hot before they could get me started. They tried me with dumbbells, small ones, you know, to gain strength, but of course they had to strap them onto my hands for me to lift them. Sometimes they strapped my hands onto a bar or something to work the machines. As the time went on the OT person realized he'd gotten me as far as he was going to be able to get me. He made a few things out of plastic sheets dipped in hot water and molded it so that I could hold something. It fit over my finger and thumbs for holding because I told them I used the computer. He gave me something like a pencil to hit keys on the computer. I was eventually able to do that.

The kitchen they had was designed for people who would be able to do their own cooking, etc. The fact that my hands did not work ruled me out of that. There's no strength in my right hand but my left hand, I finally was able to use two fingers, my index finger and my thumb on my left hand, and to this day that is still all I can use. Simple things like turning a page on a magazine I had to work with that. They had special tools for dressing. They brought in clothes that were too large and I tried to get them on. Well, I think they finally realized that was not going to be the case with me but we still practiced. I could never stand up and pull them the rest of the way; that's the problem. They gave hints that I could get my left arm into things and pull over but I could not get my right arm into anything without assistance. We practiced turning pages with my left hand because my right hand is not that usable. To make matters worse, apparently, the aides one day in bathing realized that my right arm was swollen. They told the nurse, she looked at it. I didn't even realize this swelling was going on. Later, I am in PT on a mat and in comes my doctor, it was a woman, I never saw her smile, she was very nice, but she always had a stern look on her face. The nurses or the PT people saw her enter and all said, "Oh, no!" Normally it took two PT people to help me. She came to my mat and said, "We're going to get a litter and take you up to ultrasound." I said, "Why?" She said, "Your arm is very swollen; you may have a blood clot." Now try to picture this in your mind. I had a very high neck brace on; it was never off. I don't even remember them taking it off to bathe me, to be honest. Maybe toward the end they did, but I somehow don't think they did. Ultrasound came down and put me on transfer sheets, then picked up the sheet and dragged me to the litter. I went to the ultrasound and they took me right in. There were other people waiting. I felt sorry, you know, I hated to jump ahead with them waiting. The girl that was doing the ultrasound had obviously found clotting where she could work around the neck brace. She went to her supervisor to see if she could take the neck brace off because she had already found five or six. She was worried there were more under my neck brace that could go up and go over to the aorta. It was a dangerous situation. The neck brace stayed put. As it turned out, they started me on heparin and another blood thinner. Anyway, two blood thinners. I recall they had an IV going on me and were afraid of those clots going into my lungs or heart.

For a few days, anyway, they wouldn't let them do PT. I could do certain exercises but I couldn't do anything that would use that arm. Now as time progressed my arm got bigger and they did more ultrasound and found that a large plugged vein had caused poor blood circulation to my arm. Eventually, capillaries started to form as they do in your heart when they do a bypass and supplied the blood to my arm. They didn't wrap it. They would put it high, high, high on pillows. I had my arm almost straight up in the air. One would think you would lay it down for circulation but they were putting it up, I guess for the swelling. With the heparin and other blood thinner given to me, they kept checking the blood and doing more ultrasounds, finally allowing me to return to PT.

I was there two and a half months with six hours a day in rehab. When I left, I still was not able to pull myself up to use a walker. I'll never forget: Sarah got me up and put me on a pad that rises up and down. I think she really may have had it down too low but it doesn't matter. I tried with her helping me to get up and try to get a hold of that chair but my behind felt like it weighed a ton. I could not do it. It was a disappointment to Sarah as to me. This was the last effort before leaving Brooks Rehab. I told Sarah that I would return someday walking on a walker so she could see me. I did succeed in using the walker a week later at Walton Rehab. Sarah never saw it.

My rehab continued after returning home from Walton Rehab Outpatient in Augusta, GA. It continued over the years at various places when I needed concentrated therapy of all kinds to recover from illnesses. My strength varied year to year and always responded to therapy after hospitalizations. I would say two years ago, I may have been able to walk, not the whole way but I could get out of my wheelchair and walk towards Sarah with my walker with a therapist holding onto me. I know how happy she would have been. I should have done it because it seems like this past year I haven't been exercising enough and I've had a lot of UTI's that put me in the hospital. Then every time I'm in the hospital, they send me to rehab. They've helped me a lot. They get me transferring in and out of the wheelchair and walking again after every hospitalization.

My first walk in rehab after my fall was at Walton Rehab about two weeks after returning home in Aiken,

SC. One day, I went in and they put the wheelchair up on the ramp of the parallel bars and helped me walk, as usual. After doing this a few days, one of the male PT's said, "Doris, I think you could use a walker," and so we started doing that. I could do it maybe four steps and there was always someone behind with the wheelchair and another alongside me. I eventually walked 140 feet; a really big goal was met.

As I said, my ability to walk would come and go with UTIs. I went down a couple of times but they put their knees under me as I started to go down to the floor. Once I was on the floor safely they would pick me up with a Hoyer Lift and put me back into my wheelchair. That happened actually in North Augusta Health Care, a very good rehab facility. The people are highly qualified there. I was lucky to get a PT person that appeared to be the head of the PT gym. The first day I went in there, I didn't know who this woman was. She said, "I want her first; I want that arm." Well, that arm, my right arm with lymphedema at this point of my life, that I talked about earlier, was so big; I have no idea how much it weighed but I couldn't lift it. This PT Specialist named Ms. Vicky was a lymphedema compression specialist. She mostly worked on legs. She always did the big heavy legs that you see on people. She would compression wrap them and work with them to reduce swelling. She took me into her care, and started wrapping my arm. This went on for several months; she got it down about half. It was manageable; I could lift it with no help. I have the highest regard for Ms. Vickie because I had given up on ever using my right arm and hand. The rehab places always pushed me a little more each day and with a little use of my right hand that I gained from compression therapy, I was walking fairly well with the walker...

Rehab hospitals keep working with you until they can no longer improve your condition to where you can move like you did before you got sick. At that time then, they send me home. I did this rehab process a half-dozen times a year after hospitalizations. PT really works if you do what the therapist tells you to do.

Rehab and walking were like restarting the program each time I was hospitalized. Some days I didn't make it very far; there were days for whatever reason I didn't have as much strength. I may have been on an antibiotic; I don't know, but their goal was to get me walking with the walker.

Walking again was always my main goal. When I was in my last week at Brooks Rehab Hospital, I experienced something that I never thought I would. As part of preparing me to try walking, they tried to teach me the walking gate. They put me on a gate machine that Christopher Reeves (the Superman who was a quadriplegic) foundation developed ... they had told me that if I had broken one more vertebra higher in my neck I wouldn't have been able to breathe or talk properly. I was lucky I didn't break that vertebra but poor Christopher Reeves spinal cord was severed completely. He had breathing issues. Anyway, this machine that Christopher Reeves was instrumental in designing teaches the brain the walking gate. It actually took four people to do it. One was in the back (they strapped me in a sling around my butt and crotch ... it hung from an overhead bar at the top and it was very tight and uncomfortable). I remarked to one of the therapists, "I'm so glad I'm not a man." They all laughed hysterically. It was so painful to me. They strapped me in this contraption and slung me over a treadmill. The girl behind me began counting left, right, left, right, while another girl on the left and one on the right side of me lifted my feet and stepped me over 70 steps per minute. One person in front, working the treadmill controls. They would start me out very slow and then speed me up. I tried to get my cadence so that I could walk. Because four people had to do it, the only two trained were the two who lifted my feet and they had to be available. It played them out so I don't know how long I would be on the machine but, unfortunately, it required four therapists to do the therapy so it was difficult to schedule in such a busy gym. I was only able to use it a few times but I do think it was a big help in my brain working my feet independently of each other. All of the therapy consisted of steps in progression to allow me eventually to walk with a walker and transfer in and out of my wheelchair.

I'm not sure how many times I've been back to NHC North Augusta over the years, but I would say six to eight times in some years. In the meantime, I would also do Home Healthcare PT, OT again and, again. They were all very good and brought my strength back to allow me to transfer in and out of the wheelchair.

The rehab has been the hardest part of my recovery. It's taken a lot of work. Some days I felt like I wasn't doing things right and I would get disturbed by that and almost embarrassed. Sometimes, I didn't want to go back but I still went back every day. There are many people that when they wheel them down to the rehab gym they refuse to do anything. I did everything they told me to do. As I got better and better, I felt they should spend even more time with me. There are so many things that I still can't do but I've learned to accommodate and learn how to do things in a different manner. I need to be more mobile than I am.

At Brooks Rehab Hospital a man who was so crippled, he was a paraplegic and worked his way to the point he used two canes with arm pads, and he would come by a couple of times a week and his motto was never, never, never give up. Don't ever give up. Every time he came to see me he'd say, "Now what's the word?" I'd say, "Never say never!" I also had a weekly visit by a young minister. He dove into a swimming pool, hit his head, and was paralyzed. He was a quad. He was a big guy but he had a helper dog and I saw another woman in the lab that had a helper dog. It's very interesting. She would have something around her arm or wrist and he would grab hold of it and help pull her up. It was interesting to see how they train them. He was with her constantly. The hospital allowed it because he was her dog. I never heard him bark. Anyhow, the young minister told me his story. I think he was 18 when he was paralyzed. He was strapped in his wheelchair chair, as I'd been strapped in the beginning. He touched my hand and said a prayer. He was a sweet young man. I learned that he was married and had children. He was the chaplain for the rehab hospital. Great attitude and tried to convey that to quadriplegics like myself.

You have to have a positive attitude. Accept what you can do the best you can and maybe tomorrow will be a better day. You never know. That's pretty much my theory of how I live. I don't dwell on what I can't do. I try to thank the Lord for what I can do. I have bad days. But everyone does. If I had to give any advice to anybody, especially women, it would be to maintain proper bone density. I had a test in November and had my accident in January. In November, I had a bone density and the doctor was shocked. She said, "You have lost 44% of bone density." At that moment, I knew I had to be extra careful, and I was. I quit doing some things that could have caused problems but as it turned out on the morning of January 4, 2006, I let my guard down and here we are...

Once discharged from Brooks Rehab, I had mixed feelings about coming home. How was I going to manage all those things? But my husband had the bathroom redone and some doors widened, which would help. In the hospital, I had not had to go around corners and so forth with my electric wheelchair. And so, HA HA; I left my marks everywhere in the house.

The following seven years, and to this day, I wait in the long healing process, to recover more mobility. My bladder function never returned. My husband had to empty the bladder as many times as ... five or six times a day for the remainder of 2006.

Towards the end of 2006, Dave took me to see a urologist at Shepherd Center in Atlanta in hopes of good news with a bladder function test. He performed the bladder function test and brought me to tears with the news that if my bladder had not come back by then, it will never come back. He didn't have much of a bedside manner but I guess that's the only way you can be when you have to deliver bad news.

I was shifted to home healthcare after completing Walton Rehab goals with both physical and occupational therapy. Use of the walker to transfer in and out of the wheelchair improved weekly. I had a wonderful PT gal.

She was tough. She pushed me as far as she could push me. At one time, she knew it was a little bit too much. She'd take my blood pressure and say, 'Well, that's it for the day,' after I had struggled to walk several times.

2006 will be a year I'll never forget because, in a split second, I went from being an independent, walking, shopping, working, gardening, cooking woman, taking a great deal of pride in my housekeeping, considering myself a good housekeeper, to a quadriplegic, dependent on others to do my housework, it never is the same.

Don't get me wrong. I am truly delighted with my recovery. And things could have been much worse. I placed my life in God's hands at the very moment I realized that I could not move when I fell, and He has delivered.

My family caregivers have been wonderful. And the paid caregivers, for the most part, have been very good. The ones that I've had for a long time are like family. By December 2006, I started getting bladder infections that would take a lot of strength from me even with the antibiotic. And, unfortunately, ever since then, I get them sometimes every three months. There's really no way of figuring it out.

After about three years I was on as high as fifth-generation an antibiotic, to fight infections. We're trying to fight the bladder infections ourselves by bladder flushing, using Gentamicin a compounded prescription. Dave puts it in my bladder and plugs the tube for at least an hour minimum to allow the antibiotic to work. It was ordered by Mayo Clinic. He gives them to me every night during a bladder infection and three times a week other times. It really helped control some of the UTIs. We're trying to minimize the use of IV antibiotics -- I only have one arm that I can use for IVs because my right arm got lymphedema from PICC lines. Unfortunately, they had to use the left arm for PICC line in recent years and I was always worried that it would end up like my right arm.

The blood clots occur in the vein that feeds the fluids from your arm. With that not working, it caused lymphedema, like a woman after she's had breast surgery and they have taken a lot of her lymph nodes. Unfortunately, that's another result of my fall. I now have lymphedema in that arm, my right arm, of all things. Of all the inconveniences with my fall, the most -- I've gotten used to not being able to walk because I know I can work and work and I can walk with a walker for some distance. But not being able to write has been very painful for me, because I always was a writer. And, you know, I can't send cards to friends that have lost their spouse or a family member or even birthday cards, so...I was always one to do that. And that bothers me.

But my husband, God love him, has had to take over everything. He is my 24-hours-a-day, seven-days-a-week caregiver. I've gotten so spoiled by the way he does things that when we have to get someone in to help, they don't do as good as he does.

The bladder infections still continue. And I end up in the hospital too frequently. My life in a wheelchair I must be thankful for in one way. If my neck fracture would have been one more vertebra higher I would not have been able to talk. The wheelchair has its drawbacks on vacation because you have to get a handicap room. But we have made several vacation trips to Disney and the beach. Being in a wheelchair doesn't have to have you sit home and just sit.

My plans when I first came home -- actually, before I came home, I thought I would go to talk to people that have had spinal cord injuries that have not left the hospitals yet. I could talk to them; tell them there is a world in a wheelchair. Things have gotten better. The federal government has pretty much made every establishment have wheelchair access. So that's great.

I get angry when we can't find a handicapped parking place with cars that are parked there. And if you wait long enough, you will see that they walk out and -- gingerly---get in their car and go. They may have had an injury at one time, but too many don't need those passes anymore.

I guess what I want to say -- because I did tell you that my inspiration for getting well was to try to tell someone who just experienced a spinal cord injury that there is life after the injury. Stay as busy as you can be. And I pray that you have good caregivers because that makes all the difference. You need someone that cares about you because in my case, I was so independent. I didn't need anybody to do anything for me. And now I need someone to do everything for me, even to butter my bread, to help me pick up heavy glasses when we're out eating and all those things.

But, like I say, there is life after a spinal cord injury. Good luck in your recovery. You cannot just sit there and you need to keep your muscles strong. You don't want to let them get atrophied. So, my word to you is, 'Never, say never'.

Testing the new wheelchair. It elevates as shown, tilts for boosting, raises legs in the astronaut launch position, and lays flat for a bed.

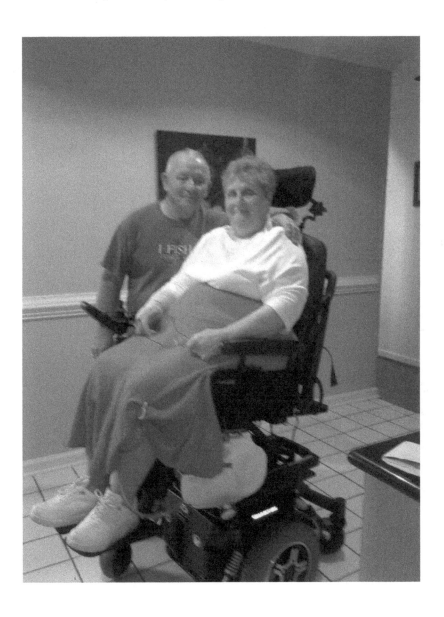

Taking a break in comfort at Disney World.

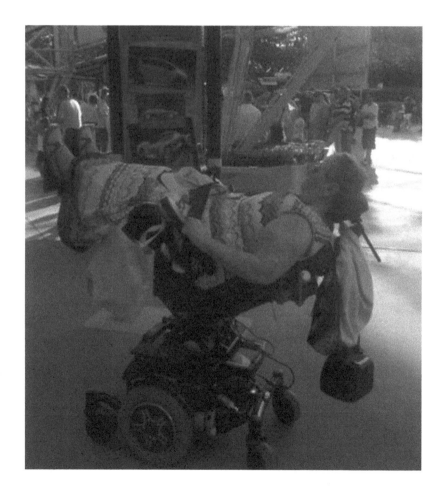

Raiding the frig

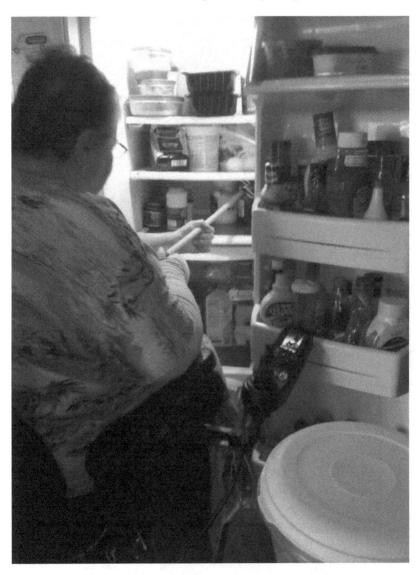

Finally back at Bridge, made possible with her new card holder – see right hand.

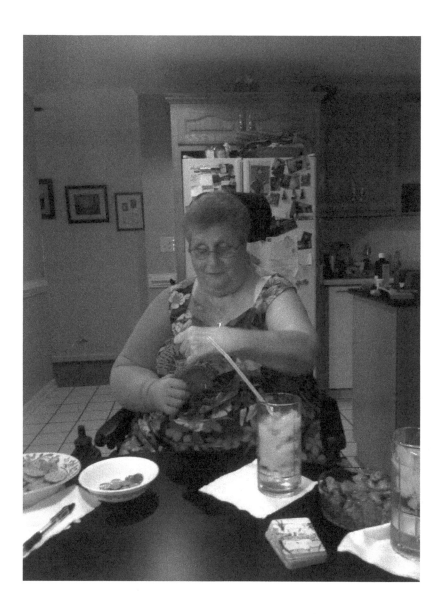

Enjoying the beach, thanks to the Marriott Barony Resort special sand dune wheelchair.

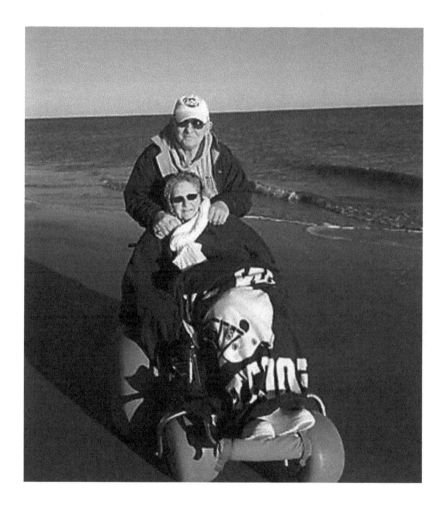

Doris staying warm at the Beach

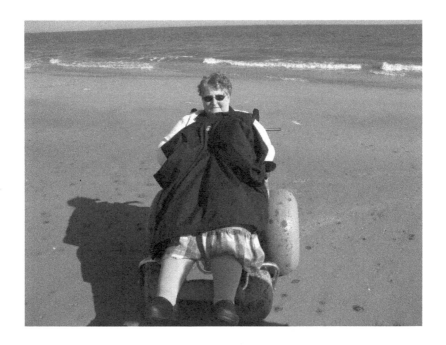

Dave & Doris at Hilton Head Beach

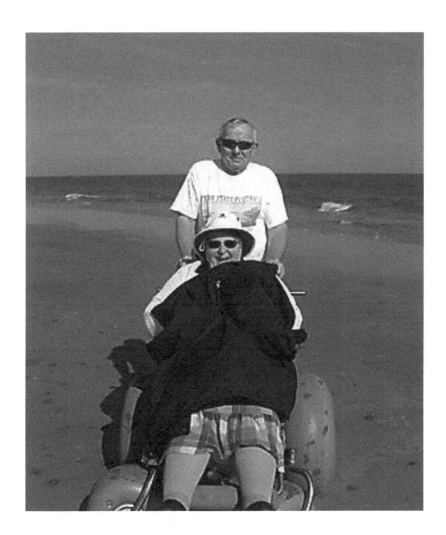

Doris relaxing in the sun at Hilton Head

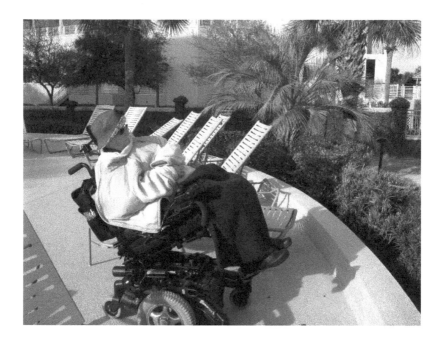

Standing and Smiling, this was our first Christmas card in recovery one year a photo with the caption "A picture is worth a Thousand Words".

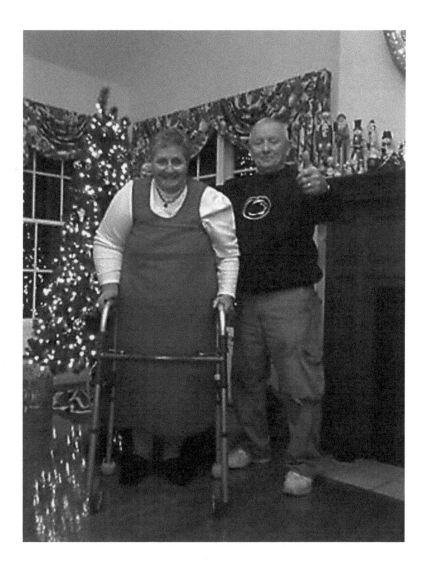

SECTION THREE

Why we wrote this book!

Since Doris' tragic spinal cord injury in 2006 she has been very concerned about warning women about the high risks of paralysis from simple falls should they have similar conditions she had in their neck or cervical spine. The concern is while she was aware of the need for surgery and certainly, the discomfort and pain she suffered from ossified posterior longitudinal ligament in her neck as early as 2003, she was never advised of the risks of a simple fall on her chin paralyzing her. Since her fall, we have met people with similar conditions, some of which did not have surgery to correct the problem. Unfortunately, the range of health status for those individuals varies significantly. But in hindsight, had Doris known the high risk of paralysis from falling on her chin as (in her case) she bent over to deadhead or pick a dead pansy in a shrub bed, she probably would have bent from the knees. Hindsight would also tell you that if she had bent from the knees to ensure that she would not fall on her face she would not be paralyzed.

We met a woman in Orange Park who had a Laminectomy and fusion of vertebra in her cervical spine who told us her surgeon indicated her condition was so critical a slap in the back could very well have paralyzed her. Another person who had the surgery, unfortunately, came out of surgery as a paraplegic suffering a risk associated with any surgery of the spine. We were asked to give that person advice and show him Doris' success in therapy. Unfortunately, he did not receive appropriate care in any way, shape, or form, and passed away within two years of having his unfortunate crippling surgery. Once, a nurse we met during an admissions procedure was visibly shaken with the sight of Doris. She shared her story of falling and obtaining a cervical spinal cord injury a few years prior. Her reaction to seeing Doris reminded her of the doctor's comment that she was a very lucky lady; she could have been paralyzed in that fall. Seeing Doris made her luck obvious.

During Doris' rehabilitation in Florida, we met individuals injured by very simple falls that could have been prevented by the simplest safety steps and approaches. We saw patients paralyzed by diseases of the spinal column causing the spinal column to swell resulting in paralysis over a short period. Those cases, fortunately, responded to antibiotics and treatment; the key is that you have to get to the right facility. I would recommend the Mayo Clinic. There are likely other clinics in the Southeast but I recommend Mayo Clinic because these patients all came from successful diagnoses and treatment at Mayo.

Doris has concerns for individuals that, as in her case, have undergone gastric bypasses or major stomach surgeries that will adversely affect calcium conversion resulting in drastic reduction in the body's calcium level. Severe calcium deficiencies will result in calcium leaching out of the bone and ossified ligaments in very fragile locations like a cervical spine. These patients should be under a doctor's care and take calcium supplements to reduce the risk of ossified ligaments. Patients with these conditions should never be in any position of falling where they could result in bending the neck backward. Please see your neurosurgeon to get his advice regarding surgical procedures to alleviate the condition.

My reasons for writing this book have to do with my observations in caring for Doris since her fall over seven and a half-year period. I would say, baby boomers, beware the world is not ready for spinal cord injuries and paralysis associated with falls similar to Doris. We live in South Carolina, a state that is in the dark ages concerning brain and spinal cord injury patients. The best programs for brain and spinal cord injuries I am aware of are in the State of Florida. Providers in the State of Florida must meet state certification qualifications when they claim to be a brain or spinal cord injury treatment facility. The State of Florida program funds costs for hospitalization, rehab, equipment and home care not covered by insurance. Fines for driving under the influence fund the costs for their program. Sheppard Center in Atlanta is the nearest rehab facility in South Carolina. South Carolina claims to be a leading retirement state; it needs to emulate Florida care for brain and spinal cord injuries.

Seeking SCI qualified medical facilities and providers will ensure the best care possible. Treatment and rehabilitation of spinal cord injury patients continue to improve. I believe one of the key messages to take from this book is that Doris' example of very positive never-say-never patient and family/caregiver attitude will provide positive results.

Medical providers cannot predict recovery from spinal cord injuries because much of it depends on the patient and their commitment to respond to therapist's rehabilitation as directed. Spinal cord injuries are all different; each classified as complete or incomplete.

Christopher Reeves was a complete spinal cord injury patient. His spinal cord was severed. We all know the life he lived following his tragic accident.

Doris' injury was classified an incomplete spinal cord injury. Compression fractures in her neck permanently damaged her central spinal cord; she also had injuries to several other nervous systems in that region of the spinal cord. Doris' spinal cord was not completely severed. Her initial condition was complete paralysis from the shoulders down. That condition, before her corrective surgery and before her physical therapy was initiated, was called a gross motor quadriplegic. The emergency room to which she was taken initiated a very critical 23-hour regimen of steroid intravenous treatment. The timing for this steroid treatment must be initiated within five hours of the injury.

The objective of massive steroid treatment is to stop the swelling of the spinal cord at the injury site. Since Doris's fall, a treatment that is more recent now includes chilling the body to also aid in a reduction or stopping the swelling of the spinal cord. We have read news reports where football players are actually walking again with chilling procedures added to recovery. The EMS personnel and police that initially loaded Doris on a stretcher for transportation to the emergency room were not qualified to deal with a spinal cord injury patient. They failed to put a neck brace on her prior to putting her on the stretcher. They simply rolled her over on her back to put her on the stretcher disregarding complete paralysis. As Doris reports, they decided to install a neck brace about five minutes from the hospital. The Orange Park Florida EMS personnel should have been trained on how to deal with a spinal cord injury patient. This was a weak link in a great program in the state of Florida for spinal cord injury patients.

Doris' multiple fractures demanded repairs at a teaching or university level hospital. The Orange Park attending neurosurgeon told me her repairs, if possible, were beyond his expertise. There is a message here. Make sure you seek out the proper hospital and a neurosurgeon for repairs. The same advice is true for rehab; again, Florida should not be a problem in locating qualified rehab facilities. Doris was transferred to Brooks Rehab Hospital in Jacksonville. A highly recommended facility. Brooks, along with a very strenuous rehab schedule, also held training sessions for patients and their loved ones. They have a great book on dealing with spinal cord injuries. I used the book often and found that they predicted and prepared me for many issues that happened to Doris after she returned home.

A very important issue that they recognized was that the typical emergency room doctors are not familiar with spinal cord patients. ER doctors do not understand issues associated with the brain and spinal cord injury patients that are unique to those patients. Brooks provides a card to patients as they leave their facility. The card states – medical emergency, this person is liable to suffer autonomic dysreflexia (exaggerated autonomic responses to stimuli if one or more of the following symptoms occur) a severe headache, nasal congestion, hypertension 180 to 300/140to160 blood pressure, Brady Cardia, blurred vision, sweating, gooseflesh, facial flushing. The card goes on to provide instructions for the doctor to examine the patient for bowel or bladder issues, examine the body for pressure irritation or stimuli triggering response. For example, an ingrown toenail can cause the symptoms in a spinal cord injury patient. Clearly, these symptoms are stroke-like symptoms or vitals that an ER doctor would normally treat for stroke or other life-threatening illnesses. My experience with Doris under these symptoms conditions was to show each attendant her Brooks AD card and provide them with home records of vitals when she was in autonomic dysreflexia. I also had a medication lowering blood pressure when it exceeded 180. I would call EMS or transport her to the emergency room immediately. The Brooks Rehab card goes on to propose a treatment scenario to reduce the blood pressure and temperature and they provide contact information for the ER doctor to call them to get instructions.

Caregivers for spinal cord injury patients must be familiar with autonomic dysreflexia, as well as know how to address it should it occur. Caregivers should go to the ER with their patients, show the ER doctor this card if they have it, or direct the treatment to ensure the doctor is aware of the patient's special needs.

To summarize, we believe this book will alert individuals with cervical spine conditions to avoid falls by taking steps to protect themselves or avoid risks that could result in an SCI. This book will help patients and caregivers for those individuals unfortunate enough to become a spinal cord injury. Hopefully, patients will better understand what they are dealing with regarding immediate treatment necessary to the recovery process. We want to emphasize that seeking out the proper neurosurgeon and type of hospital with skill level needed to effect a proper repair is essential. Locating the proper rehab facility with necessary skills for physical therapists, occupational therapists, and as necessary, speech therapists that will give the patient a much better chance for recovering to the point their injury will allow. Properly qualified SCI Rehab hospitals will prescribe the proper wheelchair for self-mobility. Recovery will vary depending upon central cord damage. That recovery can be the use of hands, wheelchair use, and even walking again under the right conditions and care.

The objective of rehab is to return to the extent allowed by spinal cord damage or the point where the patient can enjoy life even with paralysis. Proper therapy initially can provide sufficient recovery to enable life after spinal cord injury. Doris was living proof of that approach, not only after surgical repairs but dozens of times after debilitating hospitalizations from urinary tract infections.

I would hate to think where Doris would be had she fallen in our backyard in South Carolina. Bottom line is South Carolina and many states in the US should address or establish spinal cord injury programs like those in Florida. All states receive Federal money for brain and spinal cord injury care. South Carolina and likely many states use that money on Medicaid, not spinal cord patients.

Finally, with this book, we hope more spinal cord injury patients come forward to share their experiences to reduce the mystery associated with spinal cord injury. We have not had time to participate in the South Carolina Spinal Cord Injury Association. Spinal cord Medical providers cannot provide or predict recovery information for their patients. Spinal cord injuries are all different and nervous systems capable of healing take years to show progress.

Doris' story proves wrong her first rehab doctor's prediction that we would not know what would not heal or come back with therapy for two years. Over seven years later, I observed subtle motor functions returning. Doris' story also shows that age is not a limit to recovering from spinal cord injuries.

SECTION FOUR

The day our lives turned upside down

I was on the road returning from Miami when my granddaughter called to tell me grandma had fallen in the front yard and EMS was there. It was January 4, 2006. I knew she was up late the night before watching the Orange Bowl football game that I attended with son Dave and his friend John. Without any other information, all I could think was that Doris had had a stroke. I was driving. After about 15 or 20 minutes of us trying to figure out what happened to Doris, our son said, "Dad, you better pull over and let me drive." We had been on the road about two hours on our return trip to Orange Park. It was about 9 o'clock in the morning; it took us five additional hours to get to the Orange Park Hospital. As it turns out, Doris was transferred into an ER room; she was left lying in the hall all those hours in absolute agony. Unfortunately, that ER makes all patients wait in order of arrival, no preference given for most needy or urgent care patients. The neurosurgeon that was called arrived about the time I got there. His first words to Doris and me were that her neck was a mess (CT Scan results), adding that any repair possible, if it could be done at all, was beyond his capability. He said that she needed to be seen at a university level hospital. They also started an IV steroid regimen to stop the edema or swelling at her spinal cord injury (SCI) location. The surgeon told me they had to initiate steroid IV treatment within five hours of her SCI or fall in order for it to be effective. When the surgeon said that her neck was a mess, he did not explain the extent of her injury. We found out later that it involved seven vertebrae in her neck, C3 to T1.

The initial procedure for treatment of cervical spine injuries is to administer a strong intravenous steroid dosage for 23 hours and wait a few days to see if or what mobility may come back. Doris was completely paralyzed from the shoulders down with no sense of feel, no sense of touch from the shoulders down. About the third day, they asked her to move her arms. She moved them from the elbows down but couldn't tell that she did it because she had no feedback to the brain that they were moving. They then asked her to move her toes and she did so but, again, had no feedback as the toes moved. This meant that the spinal cord was not severed completely. She had central spinal cord damage as indicated by the paralysis but any movement provided hope that some sort of recovery with repair of the fractured neck region was possible.

In the following days, we watched with angst for any hint of improvement or change. At some point, nerves started firing off a nerve center located between her shoulders. She would experience jolting severe electrical shocks from that nerve center out and down both arms over the next day or so. At that time, the feeling started to come back in her upper arms first with a pressure feeling. She felt pressure to the touch. Doris knew you were touching her from her shoulders and down her arms progressively. The sensation of touch varied significantly from pressure initially to a tingling, to pain, finally to a normal sensation of touch or feeling. I remember leaving her at 10 o'clock one night in the ICU and the normal feeling was down to the elbow. When I came back the next morning she knew we were touching her down to just above the wrist. The rate of progression of feelings returning in her arms/hands slowed from days to years from that point on. Actually, over seven years later, the sense of touch in her extremities, such as the little fingers and toes never returned. Feeling in her legs never really came back to normal touch; she says they feel like logs. Feeling never really came back in her abdomen in the tummy area. Her bladder function never came back. For the sensations that did start to return, we knew we were witnessing God's miracle in Doris' body, the body He created. What an awesome witness. What was so interesting in that timeframe was that we were witnessing the body waking up to the extent that it could heal the injuries to her cervical spine.

It took until the 11th of January for the Orange Park neurosurgeon to connect with the neurosurgical team at Shands Hospital at the University of Florida in Gainesville 55 miles away. I was by Doris' side at all times. We rejoiced when the word came that they had a bed for Doris at Shands, a 695-bed trauma hospital for probably the whole Panhandle and surrounding states; an outstanding hospital. The ambulance came at 10 o'clock in the evening on January 10. I asked if I could ride in the ambulance with Doris on the trip to Gainesville. I was reminded that there were insurance issues but the EMS person relented and said okay. I was completely flabbergasted when the nurse said no when, just as we left, the driver asked the ICU nurse in charge "Were there any fractures." What followed was a ride from hell, railroad crossings, new construction the driver was hitting bumps seemingly deliberately. Finally, I said, "Look, there are fractures in her neck that paralyzed her; tell the driver to ease up on the bumps." Doris was taken off IV and given massive doses of pain meds for the trip. She felt every bump.

We finally arrived at Shands in spite of the ambulance fiasco. They were waiting for Doris. She was a direct admit. Shortly after arrival, a young doctor came in. He was the Neural team on-call doctor. The first words out of his mouth were to identify precisely the fractured ligament ossified condition as her posterior longitudinal ligament. This doctor had done his homework before we arrived. He said they had a full day of surgery booked but they would fit Doris into the schedule that day. His calming description of what had happened in Doris' neck set the tone by everyone we encountered at Shands Hospital from that point. I knew we were in the right place for Doris, still running on adrenalin but with guarded relief.

Doris was moved to the surgical floor about 5 o'clock in the evening. Surgery was scheduled for 7 PM. The Surgery waiting area was a zoo, people on litters lined up in double rows 8-10 stations long. More coming in as patients exited to OR rooms. Doris either refused or could not be given any pain meds prior to the surgery so our son and I comforted her with heat from our hands as we placed them below the base of her neck while waiting for surgery. We were obviously very concerned about how any such procedure could be performed on a patient with many fractures in her neck. Could not fathom them intubating her. It was a nightmare trying to get any comfort in the possibility of the surgery even working.

An anesthesiologist came to talk to us. He echoed our concern about this being a major surgery normally requiring that the head is moved back for intubation by inserting a tube down into her throat. He said this procedure was impossible for spinal cord injury cervical spinal patients. I don't recall his name but soon after, the attending anesthesiologist came to Doris' bedside to explain every step and every precaution he was taking to ensure all threats were addressed. He told us they used optics to intubate cervical SCI patients. I can tell you that attending anesthesiologist left us relieved with a good feeling about the surgery. He eased my worries regarding their ability to pull it off. Think about it, to perform a Laminectomy to remove bone fragments impinging on the spinal cord over seven vertebrae with many fractures over the length C3 to T1 without making her paralysis worse. They would stabilize the neck with fusion and screws over six vertebrae. We found out later that they had enough bony mass to fuse seven vertebrae. I asked the neurosurgeon how in the world could they do surgery literally in contact with the spinal cord and not, in fact, do more damage than they started with. He replied that they instrumented her brain and nervous system that responded any time they were near encroaching on the central cord and they backed off. By the grace of God, and what has to be one of the most highly skilled neurosurgical teams in the world, surgery went flawlessly. About 4 hours later, I got a call in the waiting area down in the lobby of the hospital; it was the surgeon advising me of the success without the need for blood infusion.

Following are CT Scan X-rays showing stabilizing hardware installed by the Shands Neuro Surgical team. The hardware was installed after the super delicate removal of compression fracture bone fragments embedded in the spinal cord. The stabilizing hardware are metal pins (Titanium I think) with holes at each vertebra for screws to be inserted into each side of the vertebrae to stabilize it. A truly awesome yet very effective accomplishment.

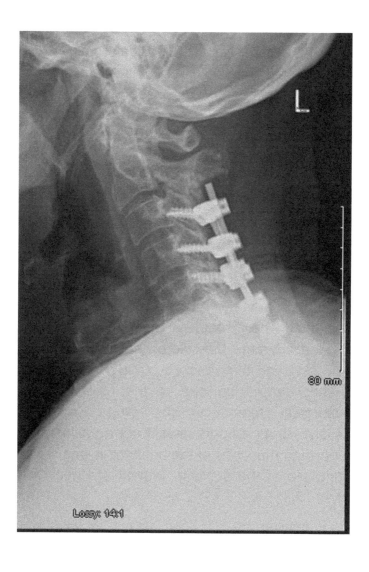

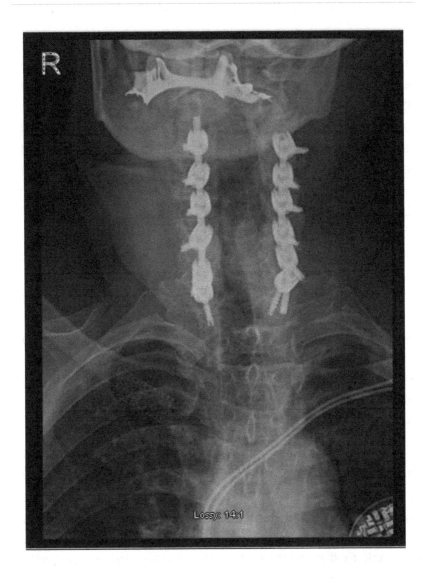

The next two weeks following surgery were just as harrowing as six days in ICU following Doris' fall. We got a completely new set of issues to deal with. There were monitors everywhere. You just couldn't get away from the alarm vitals going all over the map. I remember the second day, flat on her back, paralyzed with a neck brace on, her systolic blood pressure dropped into the low 80's. They manipulated the table and dealt with it. A highly trained nurse dealt with it, no panic, just a typical day on the job. It was a pretty dicey experience from my perspective, after all, it was the ICU. I was amazed the second day when a young lady in a wheelchair, a paraplegic showed up to assess Doris' muscle tone in her legs and arms. This physical examination assessed her overall condition as a start to Shands physical therapy (PT) program for Doris just a day after her surgery. In retrospect, this PT evaluation shows why Shands is the most highly regarded trauma hospital in the world. Back to the young lady PT evaluator ... she was paralyzed in an automobile accident as a teenager. This therapist had amazing dexterity in whipping around the bed doing a thorough examination. Shands showed, as we learned many times over the years with many hospital visits time and time again, that spinal cord injuries' physical therapy must begin immediately to keep the muscle tone from deteriorating and minimize recovery.

Watching this paraplegic do her job was just what the doctor ordered, providing some hope that recovery was in our future and assurance in knowing that Doris was in excellent care. Doris was in intensive care rooms during the first week following surgery. I left Doris' side to go back to the motel to take a shower and come back. She was in outstanding care no question about that. The level of detail that the lead surgeon directed was very reassuring at a time when you need it most. Details down to repeatedly checking the 29° angle set on the hospital bed to minimize pressure on her neck. She was moved to her third room on the same floor into the second week. At that point, they started preparing her to be stable in sitting up. The procedure was focused primarily on keeping enough blood supply to her brain when her upper body was vertical in the sitting position. They wrapped her legs and performed many attempts over three days with blood pressure stabilizing from a low of 75 to over 100. Once they got her stable in a sitting position, they brought the physical therapists in to start PT in training Doris to sit up again.

In the third week, two weeks after surgery, we had the most moving experience of that whole nightmarish time period. Doris lifted her left hand and moved her thumb and forefinger a small fraction of an inch in a pincer motion. We praised God and cried, embraced rejoicing. What happened was a very slight movement or response that was the start of Doris' neural system starting to fire again. That 3rd week was the start of what was to be one of the most amazing yet tragic periods of my life. My initial reaction in rejoicing to see those two fingers move led me to assume that Doris was on the way back to full mobility. The tragedy surfaced over the next 3 months as I came to realize Doris' motor functions had completely left her brain. It was then that we became aware of the wonderfully rewarding profession of Physical and Occupational Therapy. As a person with a scientific mind, I will never understand the phenomenon of a spinal cord injury where, in an instant, the brain's knowledge of and the brain's ability to initiate mobility disappears. I hope that someday a neurosurgeon will explain it to me.

Doris had to learn how to sit, stand, and walk to the limits constrained by permanent damage from her SCI. She was a model patient. She did everything they asked of her. It can be said that she recovered everything that was possible given the injuries to her central cord.

Her left hand was closed, claw-like. The right hand was open, not by her efforts and therapy; it was actually damaged in the middle of her rehab at Brooks Rehab by an organization that I'll discuss later. Sadly enough, the limits of her recovery regarding the hands were the severe damage to vertebrae C6 creating claw-like formation and limited use of the hands. Ossification of her cervical spine over the years with the progression of her osteoarthritis revealed itself when she started to drop things and experienced numbness in her pinky fingers. Doris' biggest concern was knowing that thousands of women with similar cervical spine conditions do not have a clue of the paralysis risks of a simple fall.

Shands Hospital discharged Doris to Brooks Rehab Hospital in Jacksonville on February 1. Her discharge from Shands was delayed a day because the heart team decided to determine why Doris fell on her chin in a shrub bed on that tragic sixth of January. They initially thought it was an irregular heartbeat causing her to blackout when she bent over to deadhead the pansy. The day before her departure the Shands Heart Team attempted to create conditions to see if she had an irregular heartbeat. That was probably the only real negative aspect of the Shands Hospital experience. Our home cardiologist was upset with the Shands Heart Team's attempted study because she was in so much trauma at the time. Doris, the trooper, never said a word of what she must have felt about what happened. One can only imagine her trauma where she is on the table, a cold table, in the heart lab undergoing a test fully awake when they decided to add an aggressive procedure. They injected her with adrenaline and her heart went into atrial fibrillation. They had to use paddles on her during the test setup to defib electric shock to get her heart back in rhythm. That, folks, is tragic. She should have never been subject to that test. It didn't matter what caused the fall, she was a gross motor quad. She was also very anxious to get to Brooks Rehab with, like me, the belief that full recovery was months away.

In my mind the Cervical Spine Neurosurgical Team at Shands University Hospital at the University of Florida, Gainesville is the center of excellence for Neurosurgery. Shands surgeons made what was an impossible surgical procedure seem routine.

SECTION FIVE

Attention Spinal Cord Injury Patients!

Proof of the ability of the brain to relearn motor functions

Let's start this discussion with my reaction when I first observed the slightest movement of Doris' left-hand thumb and forefinger.

It was two weeks after the neural team at Shands University Hospital in Gainesville, at the University of Florida performed a Laminectomy/fusion and installed titanium rods and screws to stabilize Doris' cervical spine from vertebrae C3 to T-1. Doris and I flipped out to see those two fingers move a small fraction of an inch. From that point on and through the following weeks, I realized that Doris' neuromotor functions had completely gone away. The brain had forgotten them. I desperately needed a neurosurgeon to explain how that happened. This is where I went astray on my assumptions regarding Doris' recovery starting with the slight movement of those fingers to her sitting up on the edge of the bed with the aid of three therapists. One had to be behind her to hold her in a sitting position. Wow! She could no longer sit. From that point on, her brain needed retraining in the areas of sitting and standing. She was at Shands Hospital in Gainesville three weeks, and then transferred to Brooks Rehab Hospital in Jacksonville, Florida; she was a gross motor quadriplegic. Her hands were clawed or in a closed position. I recall my reaction the first time they set her up. They asked her to lift her feet and she did so. They asked her to extend her legs and she did it. Shands Hospital initiated physical therapy (PT) from the very first day out of surgery. They were in her room daily moving her legs and performing exercises in a prone position. Key point physical therapy after a spinal cord injury should begin immediately. Once I saw this movement, and as the days progressed, I assumed that the motor functions were still there, that it was just a matter of initiating them. That assumption was completely off base. It took the next several weeks for me to come to the full realization of the fact that the brain had forgotten her neuromotor functions and would need retraining. I sent many email messages to Aiken friends and concerned folks leading them and myself to believe that Doris would return to full function.

Rehab was a slow but very energetic two times a day process. They had to develop the ability to stand and the ability to sit that took a major effort because her body first had to learn how to control blood pressure going from supine to sitting position. It took several days of short time intervals for Doris to adjust to being in a sitting position in order for the blood pressure to stay above 70 in the sitting position. When one holds a baby in a standing position so that his feet are dangling, he stomps his feet to teach the brain proprioception. Definition – an unconscious perception, the ability to sense the position and location and orientation of the body parts, which for walking is the brain knowing where in orientation the feet are at all times, something we take for granted. Once Brooks Rehab got Doris to the standing position with a strapped lift arrangement under her buttocks which allowed her elbows to rest on a table, she was asked to stomp her feet. This was to teach her brain proprioception. When she got into the next phase, where she was up on parallel bars, Doris' very experienced therapist working with her put her leg between Doris' legs as she walked to guide her legs because her feet would have crossed over each other and she would have tripped. Proprioception was a long way from re-establishing itself. Seven years later, she is more comfortable watching her feet placement as she walks and turns with the walker. Her PT therapist used to walk Doris approximately 50 feet in the house and her feet tracked very well, a great improvement from those first days on the parallel bars.

The message here is that with a spinal cord injury, recoverable neuromotor functions can be relearned with therapy. Having witnessed what Doris accomplished, which is no less than a miracle, it is certainly safe to say that the brain can relearn neuromotor functions lost in a spinal cord accident or spinal cord injury. I can recall an occupational therapy session where the therapist blindfolded Doris and then laid out three types of material in front of her. One was linoleum, a very smooth surface; the other was a medium, rough surface; and the third was an even rougher surface like a carpet. She asked Doris to identify the smoothest or roughest surfaces with her right-hand. She could not perform that function. She could not identify the difference between those three very different surfaces. She then asked Doris to do the same test with the left-hand and she identified all three surfaces correctly. Then the therapist told her to repeat with the right hand and Doris identified them all correctly. In that session, the left-hand trained the right-hand to identify the different surfaces correctly

I witnessed motor function improvement progression in the years following those first two years up to the seven years when she passed. Contrary to the initial SCI doctor's advice, Doris' motor functions through nervous systems healing process continued well beyond two years. I am amazed daily when I look at her do something like reach down to straighten her dress with her left-hand while standing with the walker. I look at these functions and remind her that she couldn't do that a year ago, six months ago, whatever the case. The bottom line is that Doris proved her original rehab doctor wrong. Nerve healing, which is very slow, and associated motor function recovery can progress for years, well beyond two years. To be clear, central cord spinal cord injuries will not heal. That explains the continued quadriplegia; for example, poor sense of feel or touch to her legs, claw-like hands, neurogenic bladder, etc.

I don't recall the exact number of units per year it takes for those nervous systems capable of healing, but I think it's only microns per year. Our granddaughter sent us a University of Colorado Medical School spinal cord injury research project that has proven that scar tissue is the major impediment to nerve healing. Hopefully, one day, minor surgery procedures can speed up SCI recovery.

Regarding Doris' recovery, one area that really is indicative of the ability of nervous systems to heal is a spinal cord injury phenomenon called autonomic dysreflexia. Brooks Rehab Hospital covered AD very well during our training while in their facility. Our instructor told us that she would not experience autonomic dysreflexia because she was an incomplete spinal cord injury patient. As a comparison, Superman Christopher Reeves was a complete spinal cord injury patient. Incomplete means the spinal cord, though not severed entirely, is permanently damaged. An interesting corollary is Doris' own experience with the repair of her central spinal cord injury: Although she had permanent damage that limited her full recovery, the neurosurgical team at Shands University repair and removal of fractured bony parts made what recovery she did have possible.

Doris was 69 years old when she fell. We had an older gentleman visit her room every evening at Brooks Rehab hospital. He would walk into the room with two canes supporting himself; my guess is that he was at least 10 years older than Doris was. He would ask her about her day in rehab. She had learned from him previously that he fell off a two-foot-high porch. His words were that he rolled off the porch, bruised his spine and was paralyzed. At Brooks Rehab, he worked his way back to walking into Doris' room to show her she could recover as well with a strong work commitment and doing what the therapists told her to do. This gentleman was her cheerleader. On his way out the door, he would turn around and say, "What's the word, Doris?" She would reply, "Never, say never!" Of course, Doris went on from that point to progress from a gross motor quadriplegic paralyzed from the shoulders down to the walking quadriplegic we enjoyed so much. Doris chose to fight back and to do everything the therapist asked her to do. Her 'never say never' commitment worked very well for this miracle lady.

December 21, 2007 (Christmas letter sent with cards 2007, two years after her SCI)

AN UPDATE ON DORIS

On January 4, it will be two years since our wonderful wife/mother and Grandma Doris was paralyzed when she fell attempting to deadhead a pansy while visiting in Florida. She bent from her waist and for some reason continued to fall into a raised shrub bed leading with her chin. Her fall resulted in compression fractures in her neck, paralyzing her from the shoulders down. Arthritis and calcium deficiency had ossified her posterior or innermost ligament supporting the cervical spine — her fall fractured that ligament several places from vertebrae C3 down to Ti, seven vertebrae overall.

We have been in 7 hospitals in the past 23 months and a dozen doctors of all disciplines tell us Doris is very fortunate to have recovered as well as she has. Surviving these past 24 months and the extent of her recovery to date is a result of Devine intervention, her hard work and dedication, and very timely and skilled medical providers. Shands Hospital at the University of Florida made a seemingly impossible neck surgery/stabilization routine. Brooks Rehab Hospital in Jacksonville took in a gross motor quadriplegic (Doris' Neuromotor functions had completely disconnected from her brain) and had her sitting, standing, and walking on parallel bars (with lots of support) in 2.5 months. Therapy at home has Doris using a walker for walking short distances and transferring to and from her wheelchair with guarded support, a major help to me in caring for her. She can stand up to 2 minutes and actually do limited knee bends, so her leg strength is improving.

Things are not all rosy here; she has had to deal with several setbacks from illnesses typical of spinal cord injury (SCI) patients. Doris actually walked 140 feet 3 times at Walton Rehab last November, the day before she got her pacemaker. Things quickly went to pot after that day with nine hospitalizations through June of this year. We almost lost her several times. She has fought back and we are happy to report no hospital stays for infections since July, thanks to the Mayo Clinic. She starts pain management treatment in 3 weeks for, of all things, an unsuccessful 2005 lumbar surgery that has caused severe 24/7 leg and hip pain. I turn her every 3-4 hours on a good night. Her bladder function has not returned; she prefers my catheterization, says that I am a good nurse. She is considered a quadriplegic because of very limited hand capability with little leg feelings and inability to walk.

Support from family, St. Thaddeus Church, friends, and the entire community continues to be overwhelming. Doris continues on prayer lists in Aiken and across the USA, and she is living testimony that prayer works. She is truly a miracle.

Doris is a model patient; she has maintained her delightful wit and positive attitude over this very difficult period. Her message to you is to bend from the knees, never lead with your chin. And to the ladies, take your calcium tablets every day. The word never is stricken from our vocabulary. We intend to prove experts wrong that claim motor and sensory functions that do not come back in 2 years after a spinal cord injury will never recover.

Doris and Dave Cowfer

SECTION SIX

Survival with a Paralyzing Spinal Cord Injury (SCI)

A "Never-say-Never" attitude is essential for any recovery and SCI patient's survival. Doris' cervical spinal cord injury resulted in complete paralysis from her shoulders down the moment she fell. Emergency SCI treatment protocol resulted in her ability to move her big toes and arms below the elbow in the hours and days following her injuries. This limited movement showed she did not have a Christopher Reeves type complete spinal cord injury. Her SCI was categorized as an "Incomplete," meaning the spinal cord in her neck was not completely severed. At the time, I rejoiced at seeing limited movement and, with the sense of feel gradually returning to her upper arms, I erroneously assumed Doris was in full recovery process. In the following 3 weeks I was living on adrenalin at her side 24/7, caught up in monitors alarming and one vitals crisis after another. With God's intervention and superb professional caregivers, Doris survived those harrowing weeks. Survival in the years and months that followed depended upon timely response to symptoms of life-threatening illnesses caused by infections, Doris' faith in God, and her never-say-never attitude.

They say no two spinal cord injuries are alike. Spinal cord injuries can make the patient wheelchair bound with loss of lung function, swallowing, bowel and bladder function to name a few. In any case, the sedentary spinal cord injury patient will encounter increased frequency of life-threatening illnesses requiring timely treatments from a professional care provider.

Increased health risks, invasive procedures for treatment of illnesses, and prescribed medications, even variations in patients healing process over time creates challenges for survival. This chapter uses Doris' experiences over 7 years 10 months as a model to illustrate how to survive with a paralyzing spinal cord injury. There are essential elements to survival that would include key caregiver timely response for emergency medical care and communication with a multitude of medical personnel. In Doris' case, permanent loss of bladder function from her SCI resulted in life-threatening emergencies starting just weeks after her fall. I took Doris anywhere necessary to get her the most expert medical care possible. We traveled to Atlanta Shepherd Center, Emory Clinic, and Jacksonville's Mayo Clinic. We also traveled 10 hours back to her Neuro Surgical Team at Shands in Gainesville, FL.

Following is a letter I wrote to Shepherd Rehab Center conveying urinary tract issues in preparation for a pending test in Atlanta.

FAX

Subject: Records Doris E. Cowfer 8/17/37 for appt. 8/30/06 Sheppard Clinic or possible office visit

Ref: Phone message PM 8/15/06

Date: 8/15/2006

To: DR G … Atten: T …
Phone Number: 404 …
Fax Number: 404 …

From: Clarence D. Cowfer
Phone Number: 803 … Cell: 803 …
Fax Number: 803 …

Comments:

Hi T …, I left a phone message for you today and thought it best to send attached medical report from 4/11/06. We have an appointment to see Dr. G. at Sheppard Rehab 8/30/06 hoping to get help for Doris from a Urologist with central cord patient experience. Doris has had no less than 12 urinary track infections since her SCI injury from a fall on 1/4/06. We are now 3 weeks since the last one, her longest time without a UTI was maybe a week since Jan. 4th. The only thing we are doing different currently is taking 6 cranberry pills a day. I am doing 24-7 intermittent caths, DRs G. (our Internist) and A. a Urologist in Aiken, SC our home has been treating her for the UTI's. Dr. G. agrees with our seeking out Dr. G. because of the lack of SCI experience for Urologists in the Aiken/Augusta area. A UTI 2 months ago was very serious when the infection spread to her kidneys and elsewhere. She required IV antibiotics to survive that one.

Interestingly enough, her bladder is very sensitive to fullness at 250-300cc, but it will not release. The 4/11 procedure attached included stretching the sphincter and it appeared to work for 6-8 weeks it has not worked for over 2 months (after a bout with a UTI) and she is becoming sore from the caths. She was on Flomax and Urecholine at the time it worked. Dr. A. took her off the Urecholine claiming he did not have much faith in the drug.

Doris' compression fractures in her neck occurred on 1/4/06, she had a C3-T1 laminectomy at Shands Hospital Univ. FL on 1/11/06. Her recovery from quadriparesis is nothing short of a miracle. If we/you can solve the bladder problems she will function again.

Thank you in advance for your support.

Clarence D. Cowfer
For Doris E. Cowfer
… Aiken, SC
803 …

We dealt with emergency room doctors from Aiken to Florida, blessed with the services of Dr. Gerald Gordon, an excellent general practitioner/infections doctor, and a dozen specialists and innumerable trauma nurses in ER's on an average of 6-8 times a year. The year 2012 was a good year with four hospitalizations. As a caregiver, you must maintain full records of your patient's illnesses, medications, and changes in the patient's condition, including resistance to medications like antibiotics for infections that will happen over time. It not only helps ER doctors in initial treatment, but may prevent sepsis if you put the ER doctor in contact with your personal infections doctor. Bottom line is the SCI patient must have an advocate to effectively communicate and manage his or her patient's needs 24/7.

See following memo to attending Dr. L. at National Health Care Rehab facility where Doris was admitted many times for rehab after debilitating hospitalizations.

1/22/2011

To: DR L.,

From: Clarence D. Cowfer (Dave)

Subject: Doris Cowfer 8/17/37 pain treatment and pain med history

Dear DR L.,

I am Doris' husband of 55 years. I am her 24/7 caregiver and my life is committed to her care and wellbeing. Doris has the following specialist caregivers in the area:

Primary care and infections – DR. G. 649-
Cardiology – DR. C. 641-
Lungs, DR. H. University Hospital 706-
Pain Management – DR. S. 706-
Spinal Cord Injury Rehab – DR. S. 706-
Neurosurgeon (in case paralysis worsens) DR. O. 706-
Vascular – DR. R. Univ. Hospital 706-
Urology – DR. M. 706-

Doris' pain sources are:
Arthritis since mid-30s (age) she has not had non-steroidal arthritic pain meds since spinal injury at Neurosurgeon's instructions because they impede neuropathic healing.

L4-L5 Lumbar pain – a July 2005 laminectomy where pain came back 10 days after. She had post-surgery round of epidurals (Dr. S.) and was pain free Oct 2005. This is Doris' major source of pain today. Pain radiates into right heel and left heel after laying in one position for over 2-3 hours. Dr. S. successfully reduced L4/L5 pain source with 3 groups of 5 epidurals in Oct/Nov 2010. Current pain meds and use of ice packs on inside of heels during early night when she complains about heel pain will do OK.

Simple fall on her chin picking a dead pansy caused Cervical spine central cord injury C3-T1 with complete paralysis shoulders down 1/6/2006. Shands University Hospital, Gainesville, FL did laminectomy her motor movement has progressed after intense physical and occupational therapy at Brooks Rehab hospital Jacksonville, FL – as you can see since then. She has fought her way back.

Ossification of posterior longitudinal ligament starting in cervical spine (compression fractures caused paralysis in 2006 fall) has progressed down her spine, DR. O. reported it was down to her bra line in 2008 This condition and resulting stenosis is a major pain source.

Medication Issues:

In past 3 months Doris transitioned from Fentanyl (150 max dose) to Methadone (up to 4/10 mg per day). Fentanyl was not satisfactory for controlling neuropathic pain. DR. S. epidurals successfully reduced lumbar pain issues to livable levels see above. DR. S. ordered Methadone because it functions more in the spinal.

Doris had very difficult adjustment to methadone. Loopyness and other cognitive issues, memory/concentration loss, etc. This was expected with 18-day half-life typical adjustment issues. She seemed to adjust OK so dosages were increased to 10mg in AM and afternoon with 20mg at bedtime.

Other med interaction was significant with loopy behavior if meds (Baclofen and Restoril) were taken together. Restoril was dropped in mid Dec. Loopy behavior continued at various levels. Methadone was decreased to 2 per day because 1) it did not eliminate L4 nerve root heel pain and 2) Doris appears to have compatibility issues with methadone.

DR G. believes narcotics intake is overriding problem causing daytime sleeping. Significant improvement in loopy behavior with reduced methadone tends to confirm that narcotics is the cause.

I have witnessed loopy behavior 30-45 minutes after administering methadone with baclofen and possibly other meds. I suggest eliminating methadone in 5mg increments over a period of time recommended by DR S. Baclofen can be reduced because Doris' spasms incidences from spinal cord injury have decreased to very few, less than 2 per month. DR S. recommends very slow reductions one med at a time to ensure proper adjustments.

See med list attached. DR G. cut Lasix (80mg in AM) and Inspra (potassium retainer) because she was dehydrated when admitted to Aiken Hospital 1/12/11. She has had some incidences of congestive heart failure since 1/2007. Lymphedema in right arm and lower leg fluid suggests a need to restart Lasix does of some sort.

Other issues:
Chronic urinary track infections with indwelling Foley catheter are ongoing issue. I perform Gentamicin flushes 3 times per week (ordered by DR I. Mayo Clinic (2007). She takes Macrobid every day (stopped by DR G. 1/12/11) that must be continued.

Please reorder Macrobid. We tried to stop Microbid 7 weeks ago and she developed UTI within a week. Another UTI a week after going off treatment for previous UTI. Noteworthy to mention these last 2 UTIs responded to oral antibiotics. UTI treatment evolved to IV 4th generation antibiotics only since first major one in 12/06. My point is Macrobid is effective.

Daytime sleeping continues to be a problem. This started with introduction of methadone. On 1/11/11, I took Doris to University Emergency Room concerned sleepiness may be due to aspiration pneumonia or UTI. After 9 hours of testing, no results identified pneumonia or other problem. ER sent her home to wait for results of blood and urine cultures. They administered a dose of IV antibiotics that seemed to improve her condition significantly. They provided a oral antibiotic prescription that I did not fill because Doris was admitted to ARMC same day. ARMC repeated cultures with no follow up action.

Right arm Deep vein thrombosis (originally caused by PIC Lines starting in 2006) and Lymphedema had a major setback on 1/11 – 1/12/11. University ER visit on 1/11 and follow up ER visit at ARMC resulted in Doris wearing sleeve and gauntlet on right arm for about 36 hours, normal wear time is about 12-14 hours per day.

Hind-site shows it was a mistake to wear the sleeve and gauntlet beyond the normal time. The arm circulation was impeded by the sleeve dramatically increasing arm swelling and a tourniquet formed at the wrist. Circulation was cut to the right hand, it turned purple color resulting to the visit to ARMC ER.

Doris and I are confident that V., NHC Healthcare Compression Therapist will restore arm swelling to enable use of the right hand again, and eventually, use of the sleeve and gauntlet. We and NHC are very fortunate to have Ms V.

She did a wonderful job compressing the right arm in 2009, an accomplishment that only qualified care providers know about. We certainly never thought it possible. Doris and I have been spreading the word since August 2009.

Thank you for your time. I will be out of town until Friday PM 1/28. My Daughter and Granddaughter will visit Doris PM daily. Amy Sharpe will be helping with Doris in the AM each day. I authorize NHC Healthcare to give Amy information to relay to me if your Nursing staff does not have time to do so. I can be reached at 803 … anytime.

Regards, Dave Cowfer

If you live in a state like Florida, care providers or medical providers, claiming to be a spinal cord injury care professional/facility, must meet strict state qualifications and maintain those qualifications for treating spinal cord patients. South Carolina is in the dark ages on care for spinal cord injuries. Any facility could hang a shingle and claim to be a spinal cord treatment facility. Shepherd Center in Atlanta is the closest qualified facility to Aiken, SC for SCI rehab like Doris was given at Brooks Rehab in Jacksonville, FL.

Autonomic Dysreflexia

For several years after Doris' SCI she suffered from a phenomenon called autonomic dysreflexia (AD), a potentially life-threatening condition that my Brooks Rehab training included in its instructions for emergency response and card-carrying instructions for ER doctors. I had to use that card many times; amazing testimony regarding how inexperienced typical ER's are in SCI patient care. In layman's terms, AD is caused by an infection that triggers a message from the brain to respond to that specific location in the body. In Doris' case, her cervical SCI prevented a response back to the brain on a mission accomplished causing the bodies vitals to go berserk. She would be visually and cognitively impaired to the extent that she would be calling my name, shouting for me to come to her when I was standing in front of her. The extreme BP and body temperatures introduce stroke risks and potential for permanent organ damage. Bladder infections causing AD caused profuse sweating above her neck fractures.

Water would literally pour off her head. Infections as simple as an ingrown toenail caused AD with Doris' temperature to spike as high as 105 degrees and her blood pressure skyrocket to as high as 230. Over 2 to 3 years her central nervous system stabilized and the autonomic dysreflexia gradually disappeared. After that time, Doris' reaction to infections shifted to near comatose type sleeps, off the wall state-of-mind conditions, and a more typical temperature elevation symptom that, when it occurred, demanded immediate ER attention to prevent life-threatening sepsis. Point being, over the years there were major changes in Doris' response to infections with time. Later on, the symptoms were more and more subtle making timely response difficult. Over the years, lung infections and bouts of congestive heart failure and increased medications further complicated Doris' fight for survival. As time passed, Doris became immune to the first 4 generations of antibiotics. The start of this scenario was revealed in the first 6 months of 2007. The first urinary tract infection (UTI) in December 2006 led to seven infections with hospitalizations through June of 2007. Each UTI was resistant to the previous UTI bacteria, a few times while she was still being administered the med for the previous infection. I thought it was the beginning of the end. With no local solution available, I took Doris to Mayo Clinic in Jacksonville. Mayo Clinic Urology doctors prescribed Gentamicin, a compounded antibiotic bladder flush that I administered nearly every day for 2007 and on a prescribed schedule since that time. The Gentamicin broke the recurring cycle of UTIs and, in my opinion, saved Doris' life. Obviously, the bladder flush did not eliminate UTIs. It did, however, manage the nuisance UTI causing bacteria. Doris averaged about six UTIs a year after mid-2007. For most recent hospitalizations for pneumonia and bladder infections, her infections doctor, Dr. Gordon, ordered combinations of 5th generation antibiotics that, by God's grace, pulled Doris through crisis after crisis.

For spinal cord injury patients suffering from paralysis, it is imperative that you seek proper medical providers immediately. Demand physical therapy within a day to maintain the best muscle condition possible. For complete paralysis, you should consider transport to Shepherd Center, or a University level facility like Shands Hospital, Gainesville, FL, University of Florida. It is critical that you reach out to hospitals and facilities that have extensive spinal cord injury treatment experience. Never give up, respond to your doctors and therapists. Accept treatment with the understanding that spinal cord injury patients' healing process is a very slow process and, over years, the paralysis condition will improve. In February 2006, we were advised that what mobility would come back would happen in 2 years. Doris' central spinal cord damage caused permanent paralysis and extreme limits in use of her hands and legs, hence her classification as a quadriplegic. I can tell you there were other nervous systems in her body that healed over time that revealed very subtle improvement in balance and dexterity and autonomic dysreflexia, as I described previously. Doris' survival was due to her professional care providers, her tremendous faith in God, enormous endurance that met every roadblock head on, and us as a team treating every day as a terminally ill cancer patient. Yes, Doris' SCI was a terminal illness that we faced head on and fought like cancer.

Bladder and Bowel management

Doris' bladder function never returned. The first year, bladder management was to manually empty the bladder up to 5-6 times a day. Brooks' Rehab nurses trained me to perform the procedure in the first week at that facility. I visited Doris 14-16 hours a day so I got the opportunity to maintain the bladder daily. When we returned to Aiken, I used sterile self-contained bags to empty the bladder from April to December. Use of diuretics to treat congestive heart failure starting in January 2007 required use of an indwelling Foley catheter from that point on. Monitoring and timely response to urinary tract Infections dominated care needs the entire time. At one point, I was advised that nothing could be done to stop them. I was at a point of complete frustration with UTIs coming continually. I sought Mayo Clinic help and they delivered with preventive antibiotic bladder flushes stopping 50% of the UTIs caused by nuisance bacteria. It saved Doris' life.

Bowel management is a key part of the Brooks Rehab Program. During the first several weeks, a nurse worked diligently to recover Doris' bowel function. I would assist to learn how to deal with what was a day-to-day process from then on. Bowel management was a major part of care and survival the remainder of her life. We learned from her autonomic dysreflexia days that her body would react to constipation from impaction, and damage to her large bowel that nearly required major surgery and recovery, that we did not want any part of.

Immobility was a challenge the entire time at Brooks. Doris had to be moved using body slings manipulated with overhead tracks. She was not issued a power wheelchair until her last day as she was discharged from Rehab Hospital. She had to be pushed in a manual wheelchair because she had no use of her hands. With digital stimulation, Doris' bowel function returned. However, bowel management was a daily care process that became more challenging over time with body fluid issues caused by the use of diuretics and complications with the use of antibiotics and pain meds. The most memorable experience at Brooks was Doris and my first test alone on a trip. We actually got in a wheelchair cab and traveled to visit our son and family for the day as part of our Brooks training process to see if we were ready to come home to South Carolina. The bowel training came in handy that day. We transferred into bed using a transfer board, did our business on a bedpan, and transferred back to the wheelchair, no problem. We were very proud of our success that day to say the least, with reassuring faith we were ready to go home to Aiken.

Infections and the neurogenic bladder

Doris came down with urinary tract infections (UTI) starting within weeks of going back home. A show stopper UTI in December 2006 with life-threatening respiratory issues changed our routine after 10 months of in-and-outs emptying the bladder 5-6 times a day. They installed an indwelling Foley catheter, changing her bladder profile, initiating existing latex allergy issues. From that time on, UTIs became Doris' biggest life-threatening problem. Early on, symptoms of UTIs were obvious and with autonomic dysreflexia were compounded with stroke-like vitals. Her blood pressure would skyrocket above 200 up to 230 and body temps would escalate to as high as 105. Use of a Foley catheter starting in January 2007 brought on a much higher level of UTIs. Bacteria like Pseudomonas colonized in the bladder causing increased health risks of UTIs. Doris' UTI resulted in less subtle symptoms after autonomic dysreflexia went away. Our response to UTIs for necessary emergency treatment over time became more demanding and highly dependent upon ER doctors' use of the antibiotics that cured the most recent UTI. Doris had that timely care because she had an Infections doctor providing input to several ERs in the GA/SC region. Bladder infections caused Doris to become resistant to several generations of antibiotics over time becoming her biggest threat to survival.

Treatment for bladder and pulmonary infections typically had to be done by intravenously. Over time her veins gave way to a Peripherally Inserted Central Catheter (PICC) line. This is a form of intravenous access that can be used for a prolonged period of time for, in Doris' case extended antibiotic therapy and blood sampling. Unfortunately, Doris' PICC Lines clotted from the very first one inserted. The clotting issues progressed into a right arm deep vein thrombosis with complications discussed later. Following is an update I sent to interested parties during a hospital stay in November 2012.

From: Dave Cowfer
Subject: Doris' Status
Date: November 5, 2012 at 12:36 PM
To: Dave Cowfer

Doris had a good day yesterday. Much improved over Saturday, could not keep her awake. The Steeler game and the iPad Word Game with the kids helped as always. The iPad from Pat and Dave and family last Christmas has been an amazing device. She is Facebooking, Tweeting, emailing, surfing the web, gaming with the loves of her life, grandkids, nieces. Her IV stick finally gave out last evening after 3 days – a record for our Doris. She has veins available and the DR seems to have decided against installing a PICC Line, a tinny tube that goes into her Brachial vein under side of her upper arm, it is inserted thru the shoulder and down a major vein just over the heart. The short story is I am against use of this procedure except for an extreme emergency, which fortunately is not the case this hospital visit, the current bug in her bladder requires IV for treatment. PICC Lines destroyed her right arm a few years ago – it is 2 times the size of her left arm on a good day, requiring 24/7 compression therapy to keep it there. Good news there is we got the arm back into her recently purchased sleep garment after 2 weeks of heavy duty compression therapy wraps. Doris has had a tough summer and fall. UTI's are on a 2-month cycle, good news we beat the last one with oral antibiotics and no hospitalization. More good news is she had outpatient breast surgery to remove a leaking milk duct, he took everything behind the whachamacollet (edited nipple) out. Not so good news is he cut thru atypical cell tissue and the Lab wants more tissue removed. It is not malignant, but a high-risk pre-cancer condition down the road.

I postponed the surgery, it was scheduled for this week at University Hospital in Augusta, the bladder did not cooperate. We decided to get a second opinion from Mayo Clinic in Jacksonville.

This is not a negative message, far from it. It is survival and we love it. Last night we were cheek-to-cheek over her chair doing Word Games on her iPad (digital scrabble) and we agreed it was a special moment. About that time her nurse, a very efficient practitioner arrived with meds and an Oxygen monitor.

She had seen a vitals report that her Oxygen saturation level was 88 earlier, about 4 points low, and wanted to check before she put her oxygen cannulas on. She dropped the monitor on the floor and went back to change the battery. When she checked her Oxygen Sat level her heart rate was 127. Now this is a patient with a low heart rate using a pacer to keep it at or above 60. It always reads 60 unless she has a fever that raises the rate 10 points per degree (I just thru that in for your future reference). Of course, it shook me up because last week her Cardiologist performed a shock and awe diuretic supplemental program that dumped over 11,000 cc of fluid in 3 days. Her legs are skinnier than ever but her potassium is dangerously low at 2.7. More tech stuff, at 2.5 potassium levels you go into atrial fibrillation sooo the 127-heart rate shook me up to say the least. Then we remembered the nurse dropped her device about 20 minutes before. A manual check showed normal heart rate. Last check her potassium was 2.9 targeting 3.5 minimum level with intake of awful oral potassium. More work to do here, obviously.

I'll close with one bit of advice. Never check into a hospital on Friday afternoon. I am bathing Doris because the hospital seemed to overlook the procedure since check-in. There were no aides on the floor Saturday. When I asked the nurse about bathing she replied she was told I was coming in. Do you think I will get a pay check? A joke of course. Doris and I both prefer me over anyone else. The message here is nurses with 15-17 patient loads and failure to call aides in, is ridiculous. BTW, the Aiken Hospital has instituted a new food program, the patient must phone in meal orders to be served. Her aide that checked her in recognized her special needs and took care of her Friday and Saturday AM. I had to call for the last 3 trays, they arrived 1-2 hours late. I can only imagine what having to ask for a tray means to a sick patient without family?

Be safe,

Dave/Skeet

Leg Spasms

For an extended period of time after Doris' UTI, she experienced leg spasms typical of SCI patients. A leg spasm is triggered by the physical movement of shifting her into bed or the wheelchair causing a nerve center trigger affecting the legs to shoot out in a rigid manner. One would think that lack of feeling in the legs would preclude her experiencing pain. My recollection of those times was painful for me to witness and show stopper intervals at best. What we were doing at the time stopped for a couple of minutes. The instructor at Brookes Rehab covered the topic with a pun claiming it would help a paraplegic put his or her pants on by simply holding the pants over their feet and the legs would shoot out; you got the picture.

Wound Prevention and Care

With the exception of leg movement, Doris could not move in bed or in her wheelchair. Skin breakdown in her buttocks and back was prevented by continual movement side to side while in bed. Skin breakdown in her wheelchair was prevented by "boosting", a process whereby she would tilt her chair back in an astronaut-like launch position, taking the weight off her butt 5 minutes out of every hour, or more as needed. Hospitals and nursing homes had orders to move Doris from one side to the other every two hours while she was in bed. Eventually, because of her immobility, she was given a variety of air mattresses in both hospitals and nursing homes. Medicare rules did not provide air mattresses at home so I purchased them for her. In fact, I purchased the latest one from her favorite rehab nursing care facility. A mattress that had longitudinal air cylinders that moved her continually side to side, enough to eliminate the need for my turning her as often. She always rested better when we started her on her good side, the left side. Air mattresses with about 16 air cylinders across the bed called low loss air mattresses had continual flow from weep holes and had a firmness adjustment but required manual side-to-side movement throughout the night.

In-home versions of low-loss air mattresses never were as comfortable for Doris. Hospital versions of these mattresses are much softer and seem to swallow her up into a very comfortable large down pillow like a plume. These mattresses do not have sheets except for a draw sheet and pad for two nurses to move her. Unfortunately, the rough nylon surface irritated her heels and caused blistering a few times when hospital staff failed to place pillows under her ankles to keep her feet off the mattress. Doris had no wounds caused by skin breakdown from pressure. She did have small wounds caused by skin-to-skin contact in the groin and by overzealous caregivers in the toileting process. Her skin was paper-like and tore very easily. We managed the skin-to-skin contact care with barrier and antifungal ointments and simple foot antifungal powder. Doris has latex allergies that presented a continual problem with the indwelling Foley catheter. We used Baza Cream antifungal and barrier cream 24/7 to minimize discomfort. We had to be vigilant in checking her groin morning and night to treat any crease redness, a precursor to open wounds. She had several wounds caused by mishaps in wheelchair transfers with improperly trained caregivers.

Doris' serious wounds were caused by latex and tape allergies in those first 2-3 weeks in ICU immediately after her spinal cord injury. That period of time was filled with failing IV's and continual shifting of central IV lines from her femoral artery to her wrists; you name it. Can you believe an ICU nurse taped a tube in her rectum to handle diarrhea from the massive steroid infusion at Orange Park Hospital? It did not work, and the latex tape caused a huge blister on her butt. In that nurse's defense, she was attempting to minimize having to move Doris before surgery at Shands to stabilize her neck fractures. In fact, she had three massive blisters from latex tape in her groin from the femoral artery IV the following week at Shands. Saving Doris' life and stabilizing her neck had priority over latex allergies in those days. Her lower arms were permanently scarred from tape tears and blisters. She did a great job managing professional caregivers on the type of tape they used but even paper tape proved a problem if left in place more than a day or two.

Doris' right arm with deep vein thrombosis and lymphedema presented unique problems discussed below.

Pain Management

Doris' pain management was a 24/7 item from years before her SCI. A failed, lower back surgery, six months before her fall and SCI, became the major source of pain late in her first year. Neuropathic pain meds (Neurontin) administered after the SCI had to be supplemented with transcutaneous electrical stimulators (TENS), pain meds, point and stick injections, to operating room atmosphere administered epidurals. All of this over 7.5 years in time. Oddly enough, her most severe pain was a referral pain from Lumbar L4 and L5 to her heels--nothing to do with her SCI. The neuropathic pain med managed SCI-related pain quite well. I will never forget we were bent on cutting back on Neurontin because it caused fluid retention. We had gone to Emory clinic for a consult on Doris' lymphedema and the first night away from home she experienced excruciating pain. We had to return to the, at that time, 2400 mg over three times a day.

The jabbing or jolting heel pain could only be handled by epidurals in the mid to late part of the 7.4 years. Doris tried every pain doctor in the Central Savannah River Area. One doctor, Dr. E. (for shit head) actually walked out of his injection room aborting the injection procedure because Doris did not tell him when she felt a sensation down her legs when he hit his spot. She was a Quad for cripes sake, with limited to no feeling in her legs. This was not the first time he injected her. In those days, good results were spotty and we know why; it was a hit or miss procedure with Dr. E. That particular day Dr. E. was in a divorce situation. Doris said he was yelling at someone on the phone as she was led back to his injection room. After unknown attempts to find his spot, he became nasty to her, gave her hell for not responding, and so she guessed on the next one and he walked out of the room. One of his aids remarked, "What do we do now?" I did not get the details of the incident until much later. Doris did not want to talk about it until we discussed the fact that the injection did not work. She could not feel the injection but the scenario and response of the staff convinced her what happened. Dr. E. is doing very well today.

A great experience with an Augusta pain management doctor who advised us that Doris was out of his expertise and recommended Dr. S., a doctor Doris had seen before her SCI. We avoided Dr. S. because his office had poor wheelchair access. Doris' pain management was solved once we could get in and out of Dr. S's. office using our own portable ramp. Wheelchair access to Dr. S's. office was still poor, at best, the last I saw it. He is without a doubt the best pain doctor in the CSRA; he injects five locations on 3-week sequenced injection procedures. His procedure deadens the nerve pain source as long as 18 months. He made Doris' life much better. Alert your podiatrist that Dr. S. can show that foot/heel pain can originate in your lumbar.

Pain management changed over time with continued ossification of Doris' Posterior Longitudinal Ligament. As a reminder, it was this condition in Doris' cervical spine that fractured causing paralysis when she fell on her chin on January 4, 2006. A few years later, Dr. O., neurosurgeon, observed the ossification had proceeded down her spine to below her bra. Since that time, the ossified condition progressed into her lumbar and changed her pain pattern to the point where she responded very well with Lidoderm transdermal patch(s) applied to the inside and bottom of her heel. Epidurals were not necessary the past 15-18 months.

The injections and, ultimately, the pain patches virtually eliminated oral pain meds. Doris was never one to take pain meds as directed every 4-6 hours. She took them on demand, an approach we were criticized for many times. She did not like how pain meds made her feel and she was more interested in proper bowel management than solving the pain. Pain meds cause constipation. Epidurals and Duragesic pain patches solved her pain issue in recent years. Oral pain meds as strong as Fentanyl injections like morphine were on her med list over time. The type and dose varied but were always the last resort. She had the best pain tolerance I ever witnessed. Rarely complained but when she did, I knew it was serious. Interesting point: In the days and weeks after her SCI, she was on a Fentanyl drip, supplemented by morphine injections. They helped her through that unbearable time of pain. Five years ago, a pain doctor ordered 100 mg of Fentanyl dissolvable tablets used by stage-four cancer patients. Doris took one pill and rejected the rest. Same for morphine. She could not tolerate it in recent hospital stays. She never liked me telling her morphine made her loopy and off the wall.

In summary, once Doris' neck repairs were healed, her pain management was an ever-changing week-to-week process driven by her inability to lie or sit in one position over 2-3 hours at a time. Doris did well with the help of some very good pain doctors and her family doctor, Dr. Gordon who rigorously managed her many meds continually for drug interaction. She also had excellent support from Aiken Publix Pharmacy that stayed on top of interactions.

Survival in Spite of some Medical Provider Errors

Doris had many doctors, OR and ER medical teams and physical, occupational and speech therapists who made her survival possible. On the other hand, she had several bad experiences with hospital staff, doctors and an Atlanta based medical equipment manufacturer that made her life a living hell. I will address the most significant of those experiences, knowing the most serious ones could have been prevented.

No Neck Brace

Doris often talked about the first moments of her tragic fall and the realization that she was completely paralyzed. She was amazed at the Orange Park EMS and Public Safety confusion and discussion regarding how to get her off her stomach and onto the board/litter. She said that finally, someone said, "Just flip her over," which is exactly what he or she did... WITHOUT FIRST PUTTING A NECK BRACE ON HER TO SECURE HER NECK. We have all seen football players carried off the field after a neck injury and witnessed the agonizing process of first securing the head and neck area. That never happened in our son's front yard in Orange Park. A team of EMS and police were there and no one knew enough to secure Doris' neck prior to flipping her off her stomach onto the litter. The ambulance ride was about 8 miles to the hospital. A few minutes out, the driver shouted back to the attendee, "We better put a neck brace on her." Her neck was a mess with compression fractures on over 6-7 vertebrae compressing her spinal central cord, paralyzing her from the neck down. During our many hospital ventures, we have seen patients paralyzed with a simple bruise to the central cord, no fractures. In 2006, those patients had a chance of walking again. In later years, those patients are very likely to walk again. It is not hard to imagine that Orange Park EMS could very well have exacerbated the permanent damage to Doris' central cord, ensuring her life in a wheelchair and quadriparesis.

Nursing Care/Rehab Facilities Not Qualified or Poorly Trained to Deal with SCI Patients

If you suffer a paralyzing spinal cord injury from a fall or surgical error, seek a certified SCI rehab hospital such as Brooks in Jacksonville or Shepherd Center in Atlanta. You should seek hospitals experienced in rehabbing a gross motor quadriplegic to some improved mobility. If you are beyond the point of initial rehab and need admittance to a care facility for rehab to recover strength after an illness, be sure to evaluate the training and experience level of that facility in transferring and handling SCI patients. Do not go on advertisements alone. We had experience with two such nursing care facilities in Aiken and in North Augusta. We visited NHC North Augusta many times over 7.5 years. One only need walk into their gym and observe the routine they do every day. NHC tailors its treatment to the patient's needs. Doris was in that facility so often they were family. On the other hand, the facility in Aiken had serious issues with training and even restrictions to staff on dealing with SCI patients. Doris' first mishap was so bizarre someone should have been fired. The incident followed proper aid in mounting the toilet. Doris would pull the wheelchair adjacent to the commode and, with help, reach over to the grab bars and pull herself up, then slide on in a sideways move. Mounting the toilet was pretty easy for her when she was in good health. Getting back into the wheelchair required assistance. This particular day, when she was ready to return to the chair, two aides showed up and instructed her to get back in the chair. She could not convince them that she could not stand herself and that she needed help to make the move. They kept demanding that she stand up and literally pull herself off the toilet onto the floor. A patient landing on the floor is an incident even for that facility. They had to call in supervision. These aides should never have responded to her call. Years later, I put Doris in that facility for a respite weekend with assurance only their SCI trained aides would care for her. On a toilet, exercise things went well in and out but transferring back into bed her nightgown caught on the wheelchair joystick and powered it into her in the middle of her transfer. The chair should have been turned off and, as matter of fact, been in a position with the controls to the outside of the bed. The aide panicked and instead of helping her back into the chair, she let Doris slide down the front of the chair, seriously bruising her entire bottom and opening a wound on her butt in the most difficult place for healing. This situation could have been prevented. There were several errors, including critical mistakes on handling the wheelchair with the patient in a precarious position. Doris' injuries could have been much worse. The message here is to evaluate the nursing care facilities in person before you admit your SCI patient. Do not rely on advertisements.

Right-Hand

Doris was about 6 weeks into rehab at Brooks when an Atlanta based medical equipment company arrived to demonstrate computer driven forearm band that when activated would activate the nerves and muscles to perform different hand functions, like reaching into a cupboard, wiping a surface, and many more. They had two patients in the trial so only the right arm device was available for Doris. What followed was initially elation when, under command, her right-hand opened fully from its quadriplegic clawed position to… what the hell… when the operator remarked "Doris' nerves are not firing yet" when her hand did not respond to the command to close. They aborted the demonstration. Nothing was said, but it took years to realize that Doris' hand would never close again. Cheryl, at MCG hand rehab, performed great work to achieve 8 pounds of grip, but she was not able to close the fingertips or hand into a fist. Any chance of even minimal use of that hand was gone forever. Unfortunately, Doris was right-handed, but in time her wrist mobility was much better than her left-hand, which remained clawed but functional in holding utensils to eat and picking up things as small as pills. To this day, I do not believe Brooks Rehab is aware of that incident. We did not realize the impact of the damage until years later. By that time, doctors had messed up the entire right arm with lymphedema or deep vein thrombosis. I never did know the identity of the Atlanta based company.

Right Arm Lymphedema

Intravenous (IV) access locations became a problem for IV antibiotics and blood labs in a matter of days at Shands University Hospital. I will never forget the agony of waiting for days for one of the two peripherally inserted central catheter (PICC) line nurses to show up in

Doris' room. Doris had contracted pneumonia and continued issues with normal procedures IV treatment were life-threatening. The wait was explained as normal schedule issues caused by just two PICC line nurses in the 695-bed trauma hospital. We were advised that the PICC line was a long-term installation, but 2 weeks after moving to Brooks Rehab, Doris' right arm started to swell. They performed an ultrasound, finding clotting, and removed the catheter. Rehab was suspended for a week on the right arm and the swelling eased.

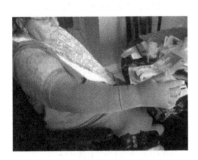 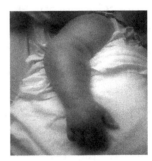

In retrospect, this incident was a red flag that surfaced again about five PICC line installations later when clotting in the vein used plugged completely resulting in the right arm swelling to 5 times its size. I realize that PICC lines were necessary to administer life-saving antibiotics, but I recall how upset the Aiken Regional Cath Lab doctor was when he learned about the situation. Seems he could have alleviated the clotting had ER doctors advised him when it first occurred. I could have intervened and asked the ER doctor to call in the Cath Lab. I took Doris to University Hospital Vein Department for a consult. They suggested a Vena bypass and referred Doris to Emory Clinic's Dr. D., the leading Atlanta Vein Surgeon. He said Vena Bypass was a solution, but not for Doris, that she was not a surgical candidate. The visit resulted only in a pat on the back for our survival efforts. Poor Doris could not sit upright, the arm became so large. We tried a lymphedema pump which was useless. It pumped fluid out but hardened tissue called protein was not affected. Lymphedema is a very dangerous illness that, if not cared for, could result in infection and loss of the arm. Interesting story: When I took Doris to Mayo Clinic in Jacksonville in late summer 2007, her arm was swollen enough to call in a Vein doctor. He looked at her arm and wrapped it with a compression wrap. He never told me to wrap it daily to prevent the massive swelling that followed. In retrospect, I believe I should have taken better care of that arm early on. What I mean is, I could have managed the arm better and pressed for an alternative to PICC lines such as a PORT. The message here is to respond to symptoms immediately. Do not let the condition develop. Unfortunately, the right arm and hand were not functional and became a 24/7 compression therapy treatment situation from that time on. Its use was limited to balance on the walker. The swelling eliminated recovery of any other function of the right hand.

In 2009, Doris was admitted to the North Augusta National Health Care Facility for rehab after a UTI hospital admission. We happened upon a staff physical therapy lab manager, Compression Specialist Ms. Vickie, that advised me to take the lymphedema pump home and "give her that right arm" for 24/7 compression wrap therapy. What followed was a miracle. Ms. Vickie reduced the arm swelling 60% over a 4-6-month period. The objective to get the arm down enough to allow for use of a compression sleeve and gauntlet similar to what breast cancer patients use was met. Doris' life much improved after that time. We became compression experts with the management of the arm from that day on. Day to day 24/7 therapy included a daytime sleeve, gauntlet, and nighttime maintenance garment. We tried three different nighttime garments and performed manual wraps but "we lost the handle" during hospitalizations or fluid setbacks. Yes, we had to go back periodically to Ms. Vickie for recovery or recharging as she called it. I never got the hang of it to replace Vickie. And she was always there as was the PT, OT, speech therapists when Doris needed them. The question is, did we evolve into a 24/7 care and life-threatening health risk that could have been prevented if the ER doctor had called Dr. R. at the Cath Lab when swelling of the arm started to get out of hand?

There was a delicate balance between daytime and nighttime compression garments. The daytime sleeves and gauntlets had a limited life. One had to be diligent, for a tourniquet affects at the wrist. The fingertips darken in color. Expect discoloration and become familiar with the patient's day-to-day skin color to be able to recognize problems. Doris' lymphedema required even wear time between daytime and nighttime garments. Nighttime garments were large thick maintenance garments with softer overall impact on the skin surface. Have your compression therapist perform manual wraps in lieu of sleeve and gauntlets as needed to maintain the proper fit of the sleeve. Replace both day and nighttime garments as recommended by the compression therapist. Unfortunately, Medicare does not cover compression garments. Congress has failed for many years to pass a Bill for Medicare coverage of lymphedema and needed compression garments.

Good hygiene is essential for the care of arm or leg with lymphedema. Infection risks are high. Cuts or wounds should be avoided. Doris had a small lesion that seemed to be impossible to cure. Impossible until we encountered an experienced a wound nurse years ago, Nurse L. We never had a problem after that time. Nurse L. at NHC North Augusta played a key role in Doris' well-being the remainder of her life.

Surgeon's Error

On June 2, 2011, Doris had surgery at Medical College of GA that was an attempt to install a Supra Pubic catheter, an alternative to her indwelling Foley catheter. It was intended to improve her life and give much-needed comfort after four and a half years of hell with an indwelling catheter from latex allergies and irritation in obviously a very sensitive area. We had requested the MCG Urology Department Chief perform the surgery, hoping his experience would enable him to identify a bladder problem with a totally destroyed urethra and over 30 bladder infections in 4.5 years. It was a Thursday. I waited anxiously alone in her room for hours. Finally, the doctor arrived with another doctor that the surgical report claimed attended the entire time of the procedure. The urology chief told me that when they opened her up (a short horizontal incision just above the pubic bone) they discovered a herniated small bowel. He added they had to bring in a general surgeon for repair and he never saw the bladder, the Supra Pubic procedure was aborted. I was disappointed but relieved thinking the surgery was not a total loss because they found a potentially dangerous condition and corrected it.

That evening I called family and close friends relaying Dr. L's. report and my interpretation of the day. I spent most of the night and returned to the hospital mid-morning to a crisis. It seemed they could not revive Doris in the morning. Her urology doctor asked the responsible floor doctor to transfer her to ICU. He refused. No one called me to advise me on the crisis. Her vitals were in the tank so bad they could not get readings. I demanded they call ICU and they transferred her immediately. Normal vitals monitor devices did not work because of low BP. An arterial tap showed acceptable vitals. Apparently, Doris' extended time on anesthesia the day before, combined with the normal meds for spasms, neuropathic pain, and sleeping pill sedated her much too much. Three days later, on Sunday, the resident that we later found had performed the surgery, told Doris they cut her small bowel by mistake. Doris replied, "That's not what R. L. told my husband."

Shortly after that, Dr. L. came to her room and told her the truth. I called the MCG Legal Department relaying the story, and the attorney was amazed, telling me they would not bill me for the surgical procedure and they would pay for my expenses incurred. He set up a meeting with me, Dr. L. and two quality representatives. The first word out of Dr. L's. mouth was that he was currently in cardiac rehab. As a cardiac bypass patient, I immediately decided to not discuss anything controversial which cost me any support from MCG Legal Department and an explanation of what really happened in that OR. The meeting prompted Dr. L. to write a report blaming Doris for the error, claiming her small bowel should not have been down there, her obesity and past surgeries set up the mistake. It was her fault. I wrote a letter to MCG Legal VP advising him of my displeasure in sending a doctor in cardiac rehab to the meeting and reiterating issues including the last abdominal surgery on Doris, causing her small bowel displacement, was by MCG Dr. M. He never responded.

I think Dr. L. is an honest man. To this day I have never received an explanation for his cover-up of the surgical error. In my opinion, he was never in the operating room. We were led to believe that he performed the surgery but the OR reported it done by a resident. My letter to the Legal Department claimed that the urology surgeon should have made the positive identity of the bladder before cutting. I told them my grandson removed a pig bladder in class for MCG Medical Illustration labs and his procedure required that he positively identify the bladder before cutting. I questioned why urology did not have the same requirement. Never got an answer.

This saga goes on and, if you can imagine, got much worse. We were now about a week from the surgery error preparing for release to go home. I looked at Doris' incision and saw what appeared to be an opening, a problem at the intersection of her two incisions. The general surgeon made a vertical incision off the middle off her initial incision; she also increased the length of the first incision. I called in the on-duty surgeon and she stuck her finger in the hole about 1.5 inches, or more, deep. We now had a wound issue that took 6 months to heal after 5 months inpatient in a wound care hospital and nursing care facility. I finished the healing treatment process at home with home health nurse. That little hole the size of a finger was enlarged by the wound care doctor to a very deep 2.5-inch three-sided triangle several times to debride dead tissue and enable treatment needed for healing. The MCG surgeon's mistake placed Doris at risk for a life-threatening infection, made her life hell for 6 months, and cost me about $10,000. Insurance had to exceed $150,000. MCG billed for the general surgeon. A friend, a Medicare auditor, told me that Medicare was starting to track hospital errors. I may inquire to see if this incident was reported. Many lessons learned here. Unfortunately, the failed SUPRA Pubic procedure caused Doris continued suffering from continual vaginal and urethra discomfort from the indwelling catheter.

Good Experiences at Very Critical Times

Don't get me wrong, we encountered hundreds of wonderful ER, hospital, and rehab facility staff. Doris' perseverance, demeanor, and our teamwork in reporting her condition, meds and our daily care adopted by everyone for her day-to-day care, won the cooperation and hearts of everyone we encountered. We are very appreciative of all of that support.

SECTION SEVEN

Doris' Final Chapter

October 13, 2013. Upon arrival in Doris' hospital room about 7 PM, she told me that Dr. G. wanted me to call him at home. Doris had been in the hospital approximately ten days for a urinary tract infection. Her stay was extended because of blood studies and cultures.

I called Dr. G. and he started the conversation with, "You've been telling me for some time something else is going on with Doris, I think I found it." He added that blood smears revealed she had an acute fast-moving leukemia. He said he didn't want to talk about details over the phone; he would meet me in her room at 7:30 the following morning, Monday the 14th.

When we met in the room on Monday morning, he said again that it was acute leukemia. He called it Acute Melogenic Leukemia, a very fast progressing cell. Doris asked, "How fast?" Dr. G. told us 1 to 2 weeks. Doris' response to that shocking prognosis was, "That's not acceptable. I have too much to do." This was so classic of Doris and indicative of her approach to roadblocks thrown at her from the spinal cord injury over the years. This strong woman simply said no, it was not going to happen. I think the interesting thing about it, after discussing it with her later, was that she had things to do. She wanted to see a great-grandchild into the world, see two granddaughters finish school, and her daughter Karen achieve goals in work. She just flat out said it was unacceptable. We naturally were in shock, tried to talk about it, didn't really believe it, and rationalized it away as a mistake.

Doris was discharged from the hospital later in the day and we decided we would wait to get a second opinion. I think, when confronted with something, something certainly this overwhelming, even though we faced many near misses with similar hospitalizations where Doris' life was threatened and she pulled through, a second opinion is the right step. Most recent was a bout with aspiration pneumonia on Memorial Day when she went into sepsis and the hospital staff wrote her off. Fortunately, a good doctor, a hospitalist, used combinations of IV antibiotics to pull Doris out of it. I questioned the hospital nurse discharging Doris with an upper respiratory rattle or congestion that she did not have when she was admitted. The discharging nurse looked at me with a cocked eye as much as saying she is dying, you idiot. I can report that we had the best summer in a long while. Doris was a long way from joining her maker.

We obviously didn't know much about the leukemia disease. We didn't know how or what she could even tolerate for treatment. It took until about noon to set up a plan for where we go next. We made some calls for references and a good family friend who is a pathologist made our search direct and successful. Following the recommendations, we decided Oncologist/Hematologist Dr. S. would be our second opinion doctor. I called him and he was able to see Doris the following Wednesday, which was two days later, in his office at University Hospital in Augusta Georgia.

When we told family and a few friends about the diagnosis and the two-week prognosis, everybody seemed to be more upset with Dr. G's. even breaking the news to us. Friends wanted to protect us from reality. Frankly, we had so many challenges in the past seven years we simply refused to accept and face the reality of the diagnosis. We decided we would wait until the oncologist made his diagnosis. We had not been around leukemia patients but knew there was a wide range of the disease in cell form and certainly in prognosis. Our appointment was in the early afternoon on Wednesday with Dr. S. His response to my question regarding the two-week prognosis was that Doris looked much too good to have only two weeks to live. He added that he would not be able to confirm the leukemia cell or even confirm if in fact, she had leukemia until he completed a bone marrow aspiration and study. Doris spoke up and said she had one of those years ago when we had a cancer scare in Pittsburgh in the 60's. Her comment brought back memories of them taking several bone marrow aspirations during that harrowing week. Fortunately, it turned out that Doris did not have cancer in the 60's but her familiarity with bone marrow aspirations and entering this scene again brought back old memories. We discussed it later and she wondered if leukemia lay dormant all of these years. At any rate, she knew what to expect from the aspiration procedure.

I will never forget the delightful conversation between Dr. S. and Doris that afternoon. The sparring between them was so funny. It was as if they had practiced the routine. He performed the aspiration in what seemed like the smallest examination room ever. Doris tilted her wheelchair back to where she was almost prone in an astronaut launch position. Dr. S. is a big man so he was able to get over the chair and do his thing. The humor screened what was obviously a stressful situation and a very tragic day: a day to remember and so typical of my Doris' many crises over the years. That was Wednesday. Dr. S. advised us that it would be the following Tuesday before he had results of the bone marrow smears. Our daughter went with us for the Tuesday appointment where Dr. S. did, in fact, confirm that Doris had acute leukemia but his lab work changed the cell type to Acute Myeloblastic Leukemia. He said that the AML prognosis was 5 to 6 months, an improvement compared to the one to two weeks of Dr. G's. prognosis. In *retrospect, the* difference in prognosis was that Dr. G. had spent over seven and a half years treating Doris for her many infections and was familiar with her bladder condition and complications to expect from it. She had colonized pseudomonas bacteria in the bladder, a life threatening bacteria if it entered the bloodstream. I believe his prognosis was influenced more by other complications or other aspects of Doris' health at the time, particularly the neurogenic bladder and the indwelling Foley catheter. The concern was how her system could deal with low white cell and platelet counts dropping to the point where her immunity to infections would be compromised. This was not good news. Continuing his discussion, Dr. S. told us that in no way could he recommend treatment, using intravenous (IV) administered chemotherapy. Doris' health was just not in any condition to tolerate IV chemo because her heart would never stand it and it would make her life much worse. But he did say that there was a palliative pill, which would be less destructive to her blood chemistry, adding he could recommend trying it. It was not a cure but it would extend her life. Chemo specifically targeted the leukemia cells in her bone marrow. Doris immediately agreed to try this palliative pill. Dr. S. described a plan to begin oral chemotherapy Friday following. There were a few things in her current blood chemistry that Dr. S. wanted to work on to get counts down that he knew would increase with the treatment. The effect would compromise her immune system, even this palliative chemo pill.

We arrived at our appointment in his office on Friday, new blood work and the urgency to target fast-acting leukemia set the treatment process in motion. The chemo pill was Gleevec: this pill is $8000 for a thirty-day prescription. Dr. S. and his staff arranged for a no-fee arrangement for the subscription through the hospital. University has an excellent program to help patients out in situations like this. Paying for the drug was a two-step process, one for the initial dose for thirty days and then another source for the subsequent prescriptions. A big thank you to Augusta's University Hospital and their pharmacy for arranging to provide Gleevec, the palliative chemo pill, for Doris.

I gave her the first dose about 2:30 PM on Friday. From the time Dr. G. had made the diagnosis and prognosis on the 13th just days into the first week, Doris's lung function or oxygen saturation levels dropped from normal breathing in the 94/95 range to 72. She would not survive at that reading without supplied oxygen full time. She had to go on full-time oxygen twenty-four hours a day in a matter of days. The most devastating symptom was her paralysis returned to where she lost function of her left-hand and arm. Since her fall, her left-hand was claw-like but she could use her thumb and forefinger as pinchers to pick up her silverware and eat. She could also pick up a water cup by the handle. She survived and treasured some level of independence with the use of her left-hand, limited as it was. I initially noticed that when she tried to raise her arm up to a certain point, the left arm would collapse and she started dropping silverware. The most frightening thing for me to witness was the effect of this terrible disease, how fast it got into her brain and central nervous system. To see her lose function of the left arm, the one limb that worked on her entire body, was devastating. I know she must have felt the same as I felt, but she did not complain. I told her, "We will help you; we will feed you; we will deal with it."

To witness the loss of the wonderful work of her neurosurgical team at Shands University Hospital in Gainesville Florida, and loss of all Doris' and her therapists' efforts working so hard to regain the mobility that she ended up with, was as tough to deal with as we experienced over seven and a half years ago. We went to bed on Friday night and I was convinced her mobility was improving, did not say anything about it. Saturday morning, we got up, bathed and dressed. Transferred Doris into her wheelchair using the Hoyer lift sling to lift her out of bed into the chair. Doris was much improved. I fed her breakfast. Doris was feeling so much better that we decided to take a break to get out of the house. Nice day, we decided to visit our grandson Jason and wife Mallory's new house. She was anxious to see the animals. She loves their dog Duke, the old English bull. We loaded her into the wheelchair access van, connected her to a bottle of oxygen at her normal dose rate. I didn't even think at that moment to check her oxygen saturation level with my O2 Sat cage but I took the extra tank and the gauge with me just in case we needed more oxygen. We get out there and before I took her out of the van, I thought I would check her O2 stats to see if we could remove her from the bottle to move around in her wheelchair. I took off the oxygen and we were sitting, visiting and playing with the dogs in the driveway. After 30 to 45 minutes, I checked her O2 stats again and they were 94. Her lung function had come back in 24 hours. She did not need supplied oxygen. A miracle: that amazing palliative chemo pill had attacked the leukemia cells in her bone marrow and her lung function came back. I also noticed she was moving her left arm. The arm was stable. It was just an amazing thing to see. It was a great visit and a wonderful day. She really enjoyed the trip.

We arrived back home, got her up to her position at the kitchen table, served dinner and rejoiced when she brought a spoon up to her mouth, no problem. What an amazing witness to the palliative chemo pill impact in just twenty-four hours. We had an appointment for follow-up blood work Monday. Chemo treatment mandated checking her blood chemistry very frequently. We started out with a dose of 600 mg of Gleevec on Friday afternoon. I gave Doris the same dose on Saturday and Sunday mornings. Sunday morning her blood sugar, a four-times a day monitoring process since April measured her blood sugar well over 200. Her diabetic care instructions on blood sugar exceeded 150, required a short-term insulin injection on a sliding scale. All day Sunday her blood sugar was rising. Doris' blood sugar went well over my prescribed sliding scale that was topped off at 200. Dr. G. ordered increases in both long and short-term insulin. No amount of insulin seemed to work. She slept a lot Sunday. Monday morning, we got up, showered and got over to an appointment at Dr. S's.

office at 11 o'clock. Doris was coherent but not able to operate her wheelchair. Dr. S's. explanation of the blood sugar skyrocketing and her current out-of-it condition was that she was extremely dehydrated. He ordered fluid IV and it failed very quickly. Hydration became a major issue. Dr. S. said he would have to put her in the hospital to install a PICC line, which is a central line, that goes indirectly into the small vena cava at the entrance to the heart. As explained earlier, a PICC line is a highly skilled procedure accessing through the brachial vein in the arm.

The Monday report on her blood chemistry showed her white count was 7200 just below the bottom of the normal range of white count, which is 9000. The Lab pulled up her count on Friday; it was out-of-sight high at 50,000. The 50,000 included the leukemia cells so her remarkable improvement in mobility and recovery in lung function was certainly that chemo pill. I lost a kid brother at 38 years of age in 1976 to lymphoma. Chuck survived 9 years with chemo. The chemo he received was very aggressive. It took days to recover from it. He suffered more from the IV chemo than he did from cancer. When you think of what that simple chemo pill did for Doris, targeting leukemia, and seeing how she responded was a witness to some incredible advances in cancer research. Unfortunately, the chemo pill and complications due to her overall health condition affected her blood sugar and no amount of insulin that I gave her could control it. By Monday night, her blood sugar was 599 and Doris was comatose.

Once we got through the initial part of the doctor's visit at 11 o'clock I gave Doris her meds because she seemed to be losing her battle to keep awake. I wanted to get the chemo pill in her including a couple other meds that I thought she really needed for the day. I held the neuropathic pain and muscle relaxing meds as instructed when she was having difficulty with consciousness. I needed to get meds in her before she went into a sugar coma. Grandson Douglas went with me that morning and we joked about how I would get those pills down without her choking in her increasingly groggy state. We laughed when I told Douglas "I'm going to have to piss her off to make sure she's awake to take these pills". As I kept agitating her to stay awake, she would come back with her jaw set, "I'm awake" getting more upset as we proceeded. We got those pills down by the grace of God. Doris had issues taking the massive numbers of pills with water. For years, we have taken pills in either applesauce or yogurt.

Unfortunately, it took all day to get that PICC line installed. Schedule issues in the Catheter Lab and one thing or another compounded by Doris' dehydration made it nearly impossible to find a vein to put it in. They sent a messenger to tell me they could not find a vein and were going to abort the procedure. I told them to exhaust all possibilities, reminding them she just had a PICC line in there a week before in Aiken Hospital. And with that, they finally got it installed. They were just about to the point where Doris had to go to an operating room for a PORT in her upper abdomen. It was late in the evening before they finally got fluids at infusion level needed. By that time, Doris was in a diabetic coma.

Monday night was a long one with nurses having to call Dr. S. many times for orders to respond to the elevated blood sugar readings. Next morning, Dr. S. moved Doris to his area on the same floor where nurses were much more familiar with vitals and the blood chemistry changes with chemo. The effects of the no chemo on Tuesday seemed to be stabilizing the blood sugar level still well over 400 and still comatose to semi-comatose conditions persisted. On Tuesday, there were times when an older nurse had a great knack for getting a response from Doris. She knew how to speak to her in a loud enough voice and Doris would move her head back and forth in response. A couple of times when she did try to talk I couldn't understand her. Her mouth was so dry or her cognitive state made it impossible. At home, Doris had a habit of closing her eyes when we bathed her, talking to her about it she would say she was not sleeping but simply closing her eyes. The interesting thing is that her blood sugar started coming back. It was below 300 late Tuesday evening. I left the hospital heading home around 10:30 PM. Daughter Karen spent the night with Doris.

I left the hospital after a request and a promise from them that they place an order for Respiratory Department to bring a BiPAP machine for Doris to help her breathe. About 6 o'clock, in the morning, my daughter called me to report that the doctor was just there and that Doris had spiked a 103-degree temperature and her blood sugars were 256. I in my stupor somehow heard the great news about the blood sugar part and missed a very important message that Doris' life was threatened and she was in kidney issues. When I arrived at the hospital, I found Doris laboring in her breathing and, to my dismay, the hospital had failed to get a BiPAP machine on her as promised. The respiratory supervisor claimed that they didn't get the order over the computer network. That was bunk. I had the nurses call respiratory, and daughter Karen had them continue to call all through the night. They never showed after my call to complain to the supervisor. She was quick to arrive. She took one look at Doris, told me to put her on her V-PAP that I took in that AM, and had the BiPAP in the room on Doris immediately. She later came in and gave me two meal tickets to the cafeteria for my trouble. Obviously, University Respiratory Department had issues. The old big BiPAP was not a respirator; it did have more airflow and a breathing rate setting that seemed to help the situation.

Dr. S. came to the room soon after I arrived, took me out in the hall to tell me he had done everything he could. Doris would not make it. He recommended not taking her to ICU, advising she was better off in her room, he could keep her more comfortable there.

The 6 o'clock blood sugar reading was 256, a big drop down from nearly 600 Monday night. I felt good about that because we had a similar incident in April in Aiken Hospital and when her blood sugar got down to 250 she woke out of the coma. I was anxious for her to wake up so we could talk about what was going on. Again, in retrospect, I was in denial of Doris' actual condition. I am sure she was fully aware of her status. At some point, she sneezed twice, a typical double sneeze, and I made the comment she was about to wake-up. Daughter Karen and granddaughter Kristin were in the room with me. I made a couple of phone calls to family and a couple of friends regarding the much-improved blood sugar level. I actually thought things were looking up. Interestingly, she kept opening her eyes, glancing at the ceiling. Karen reported she had been doing the same thing most of the night. I believe Doris was seeing the Lord and family that had passed before her. About 1 o'clock, I went over and kissed her on the forehead and told her, "Doris, you have been awake since yesterday, how about closing your eyes and get some rest, I love you." At 1:20, I looked at her and saw that she wasn't breathing. I called the Nurses station. They came to the room and confirmed she was not breathing. They called Dr. S. up from his office and he confirmed Doris had gone to be with her Lord.

Doris and I had been talking for months about every health set back we had conquered over 7.5 years, the bladder infections and pneumonia. There were a dozen in 2007 and in a good year there were 4 hospitalizations, as in 2012. By 2009, Doris had become resistant to 4 generations of antibiotics. We knew that one day she would not be able to fight off an infection. In recent months, especially with her in sepsis in May, we talked about accepting losing her to something we could not control. My fear certainly was that the bladder was going to be a major issue once her white blood cell count and platelets got down to a certain point. Her immune system would not be able to fight the colonized bacteria in her bladder. Dr. S. confirmed this scenario when I saw him a few weeks later. He said Doris did not have a chance. But what stands out through all of that is that her will and her perseverance to survive never wavered except for the complaint that the two-week prognosis was not acceptable. Her survival for nearly 8 years as a quadriplegic was purely her determination to survive and persevere regardless of the odds. I can rationalize and accept losing Doris to this vicious leukemia. Of all things, leukemia that seemed to come out of nowhere and take her away. Now after Doris passed away on October 30, 2013, I think it may have been God's way to bring her home in the least painful and least suffering manner. I say the least suffering, least painful while admitting it being impossible to describe how I felt when I saw her lose the function of that left arm and hand within 2 weeks. She and I would never have wanted her to suffer the setback into paralysis immobility that she was heading for with this leukemia.

For paralyzed SCI patients with normal bladder functions, the chance of survival with treatable Leukemia using the palliative chemo pill has to be good. I have a non-SCI friend that has been using a similar palliative pill for over 5 years now. He is doing very well. Cancer research has been incredible. My experience with losing four immediate family members to cancer and observing Doris respond to Gleevec gives me a great perspective on the marvels of modern-day cancer treatment. She certainly would have had the chance to survive with that chemo pill had she not had an indwelling Foley catheter with bacteria in the bladder.

It was a wonderful eight years. We treasured every moment, every day. We learned a lot and with this book, our hope is that we can help someone unfortunate enough to get into a similar situation. I believe more SCI patients should share their life after SCI. There are many unknowns about how to live with a paralyzing SCI, how to manage life with paralysis; manage professional caregivers and health care providers to help in survival and to get the best life possible given your circumstances. There is good in everything. If Doris' fractures had been one vertebra higher she would not have been able to breathe. She would have died there on the spot.

As Doris said, you "never say never." In recent years there have been many incidences showing that the brain can be retrained from many health setbacks, like SCI in Doris's case. Spinal cord and stroke victims are recovering motor functions with therapy like never before. The mobility functions that can be recovered are limited by the actual damage to the central cord. In Doris' case, she recovered to be able to enjoy life by retraining her brain from a gross motor quadriplegic paralyzed from the shoulders down, to walking from our front door 45 feet into the sunroom with a walker. She did it many times when she was healthy. I witnessed her improved subtle aspects of mobility and healing over 7 years. Many times, I would see her do things like grabbing the wheelchair with her arms, flinging her legs and feet straight out for me to lower her wheelchair footrests. We were experiencing mobility improvements years later. Way beyond the 2-year limit for improvements told us days after her SCI. I would come home to find her picking up "thingy," a 3-foot long gripper lying on the table. She would explain that she had to pick something up she had dropped. I would say, "When did you start that move?" Her needs for walking were to maintain her muscle tone and be able to stay on her feet long enough to transfer in and out of her wheelchair. She did wonders with that objective. I am convinced her drive to keep exercising and moving improved dexterity over the years to enable ever so small but very important mobility improvements. I will never forget seeing her half out of her wheelchair pulling up into position perfectly for mammograms the last 2 years.

Probably the most important message from Doris' experience is that she may have avoided nearly 8 years in a wheelchair if she would have bent from her knees or knelt down on her knees on the ground to deadhead that pansy on January 4, 2006. If a doctor claiming to be a neurologist would have warned her of risks of a simple fall when he diagnosed cervical spine condition in 2003, she may not have bent from her waist leading with her chin that fateful day. Clearly, the message Doris wanted to convey is that women take every precaution necessary to prevent falling on your face if you have osteoarthritis of your cervical spine.

In closing, I would offer that caring for Doris was rewarding beyond belief. Her upbeat attitude and positive view of life reinforced me day in and day out. Doris taught me to see the good in every aspect of life. I have often said Doris' tragic accident and paralysis forced us to focus on each other with no interferences 24/7 for almost eight wonderful years. I will treasure that experience to my grave.

Doris, your story is on the street as you wished it would be so others may learn from your experience.

Rest in peace, my Guardian Angel.